Update on Spine Imaging

Editor

MARIO MUTO

MAGNETIC RESONANCE IMAGING CLINICS OF NORTH AMERICA

www.mri.theclinics.com

Consulting Editors
SURESH K. MUKHERJI
LYNNE S. STEINBACH

August 2016 • Volume 24 • Number 3

ELSEVIER

1600 John F. Kennedy Boulevard • Suite 1800 • Philadelphia, Pennsylvania, 19103-2899

http://www.mri.theclinics.com

MRI CLINICS OF NORTH AMERICA Volume 24, Number 3
August 2016 ISSN 1064-9689, ISBN 13: 978-0-323-47687-4

Editor: John Vassallo (j.vassallo@elsevier.com)
Developmental Editor: Meredith Clinton

Magnetic Resonance Imaging Clinics of North America (ISSN 1064-9689) is published quarterly by Elsevier Inc., 360 Park Avenue South, New York, NY 10010-1710. Months of issue are February, May, August, and November. Business and Editorial Offices: 1600 John F. Kennedy Blvd., Ste. 1800, Philadelphia, PA 19103-2899. Customer Service Office: 3251 Riverport Lane, Maryland Heights, MO 63043. Periodicals postage paid at New York, NY and additional mailing offices. Subscription prices are $380.00 per year (domestic individuals), $636.00 per year (domestic institutions), $100.00 per year (domestic students/residents), $420.00 per year (Canadian individuals), $828.00 per year (Canadian institutions), $545.00 per year (international individuals), $828.00 per year (international institutions), and $275.00 per year (international and Canadian students/residents). International air speed delivery is included in all *Clinics* subscription prices. All prices are subject to change without notice. **POSTMASTER:** Send address changes to *Magnetic Resonance Imaging Clinics*, Elsevier Health Sciences Division, Subscription Customer Service, 3251 Riverport Lane, Maryland Heights, MO 63043. Customer Service (orders, claims, online, change of address): Elsevier Health Sciences Division, Subscription **Customer Service, 3251 Riverport Lane, Maryland Heights, MO 63043. Tel:1-800-654-2452 (U.S. and Canada); 314-447-8871 (outside U.S. and Canada). Fax: 314-447-8029. E-mail: journalscustomer service-usa@elsevier.com (for print support); journalsonlinesupport-usa@elsevier.com (for online support).**

Reprints. For copies of 100 or more of articles in this publication, please contact the Commercial Reprints Department, Elsevier Inc., 360 Park Avenue South, New York, NY 10010-1710. Tel.: 212-633-3874; Fax: 212-633-3820; E-mail: reprints@elsevier.com.

Magnetic Resonance Imaging Clinics of North America is covered in the *RSNA Index of Imaging Literature, MEDLINE/PubMed (Index Medicus),* and *EMBASE/Excerpta Medica.*

Contributors

CONSULTING EDITORS

SURESH K. MUKHERJI, MD, MBA, FACR
Department of Radiology, Michigan State
University, East Lansing, Michigan

LYNNE S. STEINBACH, MD, FACR
Professor of Radiology and Orthopaedic
Surgery, Department of Radiology and
Biomedical Imaging, University of California
San Francisco, San Francisco, California

EDITOR

MARIO MUTO, MD
Chairman, Neuroradiology Department,
Cardarelli Hospital, Naples, Italy

AUTHORS

TITO BASSANI, PhD
Laboratory of Biological Structures Mechanics,
IRCCS Istituto Ortopedico Galeazzi, Milan, Italy

MATTEO BELLINI, MD
Neuroimaging and Neurointerventional Unit,
Department of Neurological and
Neurosensorial Sciences, General Hospital
"Santa Maria alle Scotte", Siena, Italy

PEGGY BIENVENOT, MD
Department of Diagnostic and Functional
Neuroradiology, Pitié-Salpêtrière Hospital,
Paris, France

MARCO BRAYDA-BRUNO, MD
Department of Spine Surgery III, IRCCS Istituto
Ortopedico Galeazzi, Milan, Italy

ALFONSO CERASE, MD
Neuroimaging and Neurointerventional Unit,
Department of Neurological and
Neurosensorial Sciences, General Hospital
"Santa Maria alle Scotte", Siena, Italy

JACQUES CHIRAS, MD
Department of Interventional Neuroradiology,
Pitié-Salpêtrière Hospital; Paris VI University,
Pierre et Marie Curie, Paris, France

ALESSANDRO CIANFONI, MD
Department of Neuroradiology, Neurocenter of
Southern Switzerland, Lugano, Switzerland

FRÉDÉRIC CLARENÇON, MD, PhD
Department of Interventional Neuroradiology,
Pitié-Salpêtrière Hospital; Paris VI University,
Pierre et Marie Curie, Paris, France

ÉVELYNE CORMIER, MD
Department of Interventional Neuroradiology,
Pitié-Salpêtrière Hospital, Paris, France

**PETER COWLEY, MBBS (Lon), BA Oxon,
MRCP, FRCR**
Clinical Lead Interventional Neuroradiology
Consultant, National Hospital for Neurology
and Neurosurgery, Neuroimaging Analysis
Centre, UCLH, London, United Kingdom

ALVARO DIANO, MD
Neuroradiology Department, Cardarelli
Hospital, Naples, Italy

MARCO FERRARA, MD
Neuroimaging and Neurointerventional Unit,
Department of Neurological and
Neurosensorial Sciences, General Hospital
"Santa Maria alle Scotte", Siena, Italy

FABIO GALBUSERA, PhD
Laboratory of Biological Structures Mechanics, IRCCS Istituto Ortopedico Galeazzi, Milan, Italy

FRANCESCO GIURAZZA, MD
Radiology Department, Università Campus Bio-Medico di Roma, Rome, Italy

ROBERTO GRASSI, MD
Department of Radiology, Second University of Naples, Naples, Italy

IRENE GRAZZINI, MD
Section of Radiological Sciences, Department of Medical, Surgical and NeuroSciences, University of Siena, Siena, Italy

GIANLUIGI GUARNIERI, MD
Neuroradiology Department, Cardarelli Hospital, Naples, Italy

FRANCESCA IACOBELLIS, MD
Department of Radiology, Second University of Naples, Naples, Italy

ROBERTO IZZO, MD
Neuroradiology Department, Cardarelli Hospital, Naples, Italy

BRUNO LAW-YE, MD
Department of Diagnostic and Functional Neuroradiology, Pitié-Salpêtrière Hospital; Paris VI University, Pierre et Marie Curie, Paris, France

ALESSIO LOVI, MD
Department of Spine Surgery III, IRCCS Istituto Ortopedico Galeazzi, Milan, Italy

CAROLA MARTINETTI, MD
Neuroradiology Unit, Istituto Giannina Gaslini, Genova, Italy

ZULEJHA MERHEMIC, MD, PhD
Assistant Professor of Radiology, Policlinic Sunce-Agram, University of Sarajevo, Sarajevo, Bosnia & Herzegovina

GIOVANNI MORANA, MD, PhD
Neuroradiology Unit, Istituto Giannina Gaslini, Genova, Italy

MARIO MUTO, MD
Chairman, Neuroradiology Department, Cardarelli Hospital, Naples, Italy

ELENA PRODI, MD
Department of Neuroradiology, Neurocenter of Southern Switzerland, Lugano, Switzerland

ANDREA ROSSI, MD
Neuroradiology Unit, Istituto Giannina Gaslini, Genova, Italy

MARIASAVINA SEVERINO, MD
Neuroradiology Unit, Istituto Giannina Gaslini, Genova, Italy

TATJANA STOSIC-OPINCAL, MD, PhD
Director of Radiology Department, General Hospital Euromedik, Professor of Radiology, University of Belgrade, Belgrade, Serbia

MAJDA M. THURNHER, MD
Associate Professor of Radiology, Department of Biomedical Imaging and Image-Guided Therapy, Medical University Vienna, Vienna, Austria

DOMENICO TORTORA, MD
Neuroradiology Unit, Istituto Giannina Gaslini, Genova, Italy

MARC-ANDRÉ WEBER, MD, MSc
Diagnostic and Interventional Radiology, University Hospital Heidelberg, Heidelberg, Germany

MARCEL WOLF, MD
Neuroradiology, University Hospital Heidelberg, Heidelberg, Germany

Contents

> The human spine is a complex biomechanical system composed of multiple articular structures controlled by muscles. Spine diseases are frequently related to a loss of stability. Dedicated imaging protocols have been developed to evaluate spinal instability. Dynamic radiography with lumbar flexion-extension is used most often; however, in traumatic instability, computerized tomography provides better diagnostic accuracy for fracture detection. Novel technology improvements allow acquisition of dynamic MRI with axial load or upright standing techniques to simulate a more pathologic condition compared with conventional supine scans. This article reviews the basic concepts of spinal instability and describes the role of different imaging techniques in its assessment.

> Degenerative disease of the spine is a leading cause of back pain and radiculopathy, and is a frequent indication for spine MR imaging. Disc degeneration, disc protrusion/herniation, discarhtrosis, spinal canal stenosis, and facet joint arthrosis, as well as interspinous processes arthrosis, may require an MR imaging workup. This review presents the MR imaging patterns of these diseases and describes the benefit of the MR imaging in these indications compared with the other imaging modalities like plain radiographs or computed tomography scan.

> Advances in MR imaging technologies, as well as the widening of their availability, boosted their use in the diagnosis of spinal disorders and in the preoperative planning of spine surgeries. However, the most consolidated approach to the assessment of adult patients with spinal disorders is based on the analysis of full standing radiographs (posteroanterior and laterolateral views). In this article, the radiographic spinal and pelvic parameters, which have relevance in the clinical management of adults with spinal disorders, are summarized.

> Spinal stenosis is common and presents in a variety of forms. Symptomatic lumbar stenosis occurs in approximately 10% of the population and cervical stenosis in 9%

over age 70. Imaging is central to the management decision process and first-choice MR imaging may be substituted with CT and CT myelography. A review of the literature is presented with particular emphasis on the clinical-radiologic correlation in both neurogenic intermittent claudication and cervical spondylotic myelopathy. Advanced techniques promise improvements, particularly with radicular compressive lesions, but remain underutilized in routine clinical practice.

Neuroimaging of the Traumatic Spine

Marcel Wolf and Marc-André Weber

The article summarizes classification schemes of spinal trauma and rules to decide on proper imaging modality after a spinal trauma. High-risk factors that recommend imaging are, for instance, age 65 years or older, a dangerous trauma mechanism, and paresthesia in the extremities. More recent classification schemes include evaluation of the posterior ligamentous complex, for which MR imaging is the best modality, and to give therapeutic recommendations for conservative or surgical management. MR imaging is the imaging method of choice when spinal cord injury, cord compression, or ligamentous injury is suspected. MR imaging is the method of choice to depict epidural or intramedullary hemorrhage and sequelae of spinal trauma.

Neuroimaging of Spinal Tumors

Zulejha Merhemic, Tatjana Stosic-Opincal, and Majda M. Thurnher

Intradural tumors are relatively rare neoplasms; however, when unrecognized in a timely manner, they can result in serious deficits and disability. These tumors lack obvious clinical symptoms until compression of the cord or neurologic deficits occur. The most common intramedullary lesions are ependymomas, astrocytomas, and hemangioblastomas. Meningiomas and nerve sheath tumors (schwannomas and neurofibromas) comprise most intradural-extramedullary tumors. Less common tumors are hemangiopericytoma, paraganglioma, melanocytoma, melanoma, metastases, and lymphoma. MR imaging is the imaging method of choice, helpful for localization and characterization of these lesions before treatment and for follow-up after treatment.

Imaging in Spondylodiskitis

Elena Prodi, Roberto Grassi, Francesca Iacobellis, and Alessandro Cianfoni

Infections of the spine may involve different anatomic compartments, including intervertebral disks, vertebral bone, paraspinal soft tissues, epidural space, meninges, and spinal cord. This article focuses on the role of imaging in diagnosis and follow-up of infections of the intervertebral disk and vertebral bone, named respectively diskitis and spondylitis or vertebral osteomyelitis. Often, at the time of diagnosis, the infection already involves both structures; therefore the process is referred as spondylodiskitis. The discussion is extended to infections of paraspinal soft tissues and epidural space, which are commonly associated. Mention is made to the role of imaging in guiding minimally invasive biopsies of the spine in such conditions.

Neuroimaging of the Postoperative Spine

Matteo Bellini, Marco Ferrara, Irene Grazzini, and Alfonso Cerase

Operative treatments of the spine are becoming increasingly more common for the availability of a wide range of surgical and minimally invasive procedures.

MR imaging allows for excellent evaluation of both normal and abnormal findings in the postoperative spine. This article provides the basic tools to evaluate complications after different operative procedures and offers an overview on the main topics a radiologist may encounter during his or her professional carrier.

Understanding the developmental features of the pediatric spine and spinal cord, including embryologic steps and subsequent growth of the osteocartilaginous spine and contents is necessary for interpretation of the pathologic events that may affect the pediatric spine. MR imaging plays a crucial role in the diagnostic evaluation of patients suspected of harboring spinal abnormalities, whereas computed tomography and ultrasonography play a more limited, complementary role. This article discusses the embryologic and developmental anatomy features of the spine and spinal cord, together with some technical points and pitfalls, and the most common indications for pediatric spinal MR imaging.

MAGNETIC RESONANCE IMAGING CLINICS OF NORTH AMERICA

ISSUE OF RELATED INTEREST

Neuroimaging Clinics of North America, May 2015 (Vol. 25, No. 2)
Spinal Infections
E. Turgut Tali, *Editor*
Available at: www.neuroimaging.theclinics.com

VISIT THE CLINICS ONLINE!
Access your subscription at:
www.theclinics.com

PROGRAM OBJECTIVE
The goal of *Magnetic Resonance Imaging Clinics of North America* is to keep practicing physicians up to date with current clinical practice by providing timely articles reviewing the state of the art in patient care.

TARGET AUDIENCE
All practicing physicians and healthcare professionals who provide patient care utilizing findings from Magnetic Resonance Imaging.

LEARNING OBJECTIVES
Upon completion of this activity, participants will be able to:
1. Review neuroimaging techniques for the degenerative spine.
2. Discuss neuroimaging in the traumatic and unstable spine.
3. Recognize approaches to neuroimaging in disorders such as spinal tumors, spondylodiscitis, and spinal canal stenosis, among others.

ACCREDITATION
The Elsevier Office of Continuing Medical Education (EOCME) is accredited by the Accreditation Council for Continuing Medical Education (ACCME) to provide continuing medical education for physicians.

The EOCME designates this enduring material for a maximum of 15 *AMA PRA Category 1 Credit*(s)™. Physicians should claim only the credit commensurate with the extent of their participation in the activity.

All other health care professionals requesting continuing education credit for this enduring material will be issued a certificate of participation.

DISCLOSURE OF CONFLICTS OF INTEREST
The EOCME assesses conflict of interest with its instructors, faculty, planners, and other individuals who are in a position to control the content of CME activities. All relevant conflicts of interest that are identified are thoroughly vetted by EOCME for fair balance, scientific objectivity, and patient care recommendations. EOCME is committed to providing its learners with CME activities that promote improvements or quality in healthcare and not a specific proprietary business or a commercial interest.

The planning committee, staff, authors and editors listed below have identified no financial relationships or relationships to products or devices they or their spouse/life partner have with commercial interest related to the content of this CME activity:
Tito Bassani, PhD; Matteo Bellini, MD; Peggy Bienvenot, MD; Marco Brayda-Bruno, MD; Alfonso Cerase, MD; Jacques Chiras, MD; Alessandro Cianfoni, MD; Frédéric Clarençon, MD, PhD; Évelyne Cormier, MD; Peter Cowley, MBBS (Lon), BA Oxon, MRCP, FRCR; Alvaro Diano, MD; Marco Ferrara, MD; Fabio Galbusera, PhD; Francesco Giurazza, MD; Roberto Grassi, MD; Irene Grazzini, MD; Gianluigi Guarnieri, MD; Francesca Iacobellis, MD; Roberto Izzo, MD; Bruno Law-Ye, MD; Alessio Lovi, MD; Carola Martinetti, MD; Zulejha Merhemic, MD, PhD; Giovanni Morana, MD, PhD; Suresh K. Mukherji, MD, MBA, FACR; Mario Muto, MD; Elena Prodi, MD; Andrea Rossi, MD; Erin Scheckenbach; Mariasavina Severino, MD; Tatjana Stosic-Opincal, MD, PhD; Karthik Subramaniam; Domenico Tortora, MD; John Vassallo; Marc-André Weber, MD, MSc; Marcel Wolf, MD.

The planning committee, staff, authors and editors listed below have identified financial relationships or relationships to products or devices they or their spouse/life partner have with commercial interest related to the content of this CME activity:
Majda M. Thurnher, MD is a consultant/advisor for Guerbet Group, and receives roylaties/patents from Amyrsis, Inc.

UNAPPROVED/OFF-LABEL USE DISCLOSURE
The EOCME requires CME faculty to disclose to the participants:
1. When products or procedures being discussed are off-label, unlabelled, experimental, and/or investigational (not US Food and Drug Administration [FDA] approved); and
2. Any limitations on the information presented, such as data that are preliminary or that represent ongoing research, interim analyses, and/or unsupported opinions. Faculty may discuss information about pharmaceutical agents that is outside of FDA-approved labelling. This information is intended solely for CME and is not intended to promote off-label use of these medications. If you have any questions, contact the medical affairs department of the manufacturer for the most recent prescribing information.

TO ENROLL
To enroll in the *Magnetic Resonance Imaging Clinics of North America* Continuing Medical Education program, call customer service at 1-800-654-2452 or sign up online at http://www.theclinics.com/home/cme. The CME program is available to subscribers for an additional annual fee of USD 250.

METHOD OF PARTICIPATION

In order to claim credit, participants must complete the following:
1. Complete enrolment as indicated above.
2. Read the activity.
3. Complete the CME Test and Evaluation. Participants must achieve a score of 70% on the test. All CME Tests and Evaluations must be completed online.

CME INQUIRIES/SPECIAL NEEDS

For all CME inquiries or special needs, please contact elsevierCME@elsevier.com.

Foreword

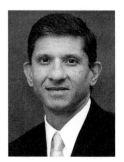

Suresh K. Mukherji, MD, MBA, FACR
Consulting Editor

MR imaging of the spine has been a stalwart of neuroimaging since the inception of clinical MR imaging in the late 1980s. I still remember hanging stacks of films (!) when I was a resident. For me, Spine MR was cumbersome and routine, but also helped identify certain diseases that could be easily and effectively treated. Fast-forward 25 years, and this author, my father, and my daughter all underwent laminectomies for disc herniations! In fact, my daughter claims the only thing I gave her in life was a bad back!! ☺

Dr Mario Muto has done a masterful job of editing this issue of *Magnetic Resonance Imaging Clinics of North America* on MR imaging of the spine. This issue has articles on the common disorders such as degenerative disease but also tackles the more complex subjects such as neoplasms, infections, trauma, and spinal instability. He also has dedicated articles on the postoperative and pediatric spine.

Dr Muto's contributors are world-renowned. They have done a wonderful job of creating a concise yet pragmatically comprehensive issue that incorporates the latest information on this common, yet very complex topic. I strongly recommend this issue to all radiologists who interpret spine imaging, and I thank Dr Muto and all of the article authors for their excellent contributions to this special issue.

Suresh K. Mukherji, MD, MBA, FACR
Department of Radiology
Michigan State University
846 Service Road
East Lansing, MI 48824, USA

E-mail address:
mukherji@rad.msu.edu

Magn Reson Imaging Clin N Am 24 (2016) xi
http://dx.doi.org/10.1016/j.mric.2016.05.002
1064-9689/16/$ – see front matter © 2016 Published by Elsevier Inc.

Preface

MR Imaging of the Spine: Where Are We Now?

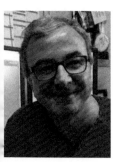

Mario Muto, MD

Editor

Spine pathologies are more and more frequently encountered in daily clinical practice, especially in western countries. The reason for this increase is twofold: sedentary lifestyle and elongation of life expectancy. The technological progresses in the field of radiological imaging have allowed us to obtain early and precise diagnosis of spine diseases, especially thanks to the introduction and spread of MR Imaging in the radiological departments worldwide; this has also permitted a better comprehension of the physiopathologic mechanisms behind multiple spine diseases, even with dynamic and functional studies.

The purpose of this special issue is to approach the different fields of the spine pathology more frequently observed in the clinical practice, according to the last MR Imaging improvements explained by subject matter experts; all efforts have been provided to integrate the clinical aspects with the more updated imaging protocols in order to associate images to patient clinics. At the end of each article, take-home points are provided to summarize the main contents.

This issue starts with the neuroimaging of spinal instabilities, with Muto and colleagues reviewing the anatomical principles of stability and the basic concepts of spinal instability and describing the role of the different imaging techniques, both conventional and dynamic.

The second article by Clarençon and colleagues and the third article by Galbusera and colleagues approach extensively the wide theme of the degenerative spine disorders, reporting the MR Imaging patterns and the radiographic spinal and pelvic parameters that have relevance in the clinical management of adults with spinal disorders; in this section is analyzed also the crucial role of imaging when planning surgery on a degenerated spine.

The variety of forms of spinal stenosis is faced in the article by Cowley by reviewing the literature with particular emphasis on the clinic-radiological correlation in both neurogenic intermittent claudication and cervical spondylotic myelopathy.

The article by Wolf and Weber summarizes the current classification schemes of spinal trauma and rules to decide pon the proper imaging modality after a spinal trauma, while the article by Merhemic and colleagues discusses the role of MR Imaging to localize and characterize spine tumors before treatment as well as for follow-up after treatment.

The different anatomical compartments that can be involved by infections of the spine, including intervertebral discs, vertebral bone, paraspinal soft tissues, epidural space, meninges, and spinal cord, are analyzed together with the role of imaging in diagnosis and follow-up in the article by Prodi and colleagues.

Because the operative treatments of the spine are becoming increasingly more common for the availability of a wide range of surgical and minimally invasive procedures, a whole article , written by Bellini and colleagues, is dedicated to the role of MR Imaging for the evaluation of both normal and abnormal findings in the postoperative spine.

Magn Reson Imaging Clin N Am 24 (2016) xiii–xiv
http://dx.doi.org/10.1016/j.mric.2016.05.001
1064-9689/16/$ – see front matter © 2016 Published by Elsevier Inc.

mri.theclinics.com

Finally, a basic primer on the embryologic and developmental anatomy features of the spine and spinal cord is provided in the article by Rossi and colleagues together with a few technical points and pitfalls, as well as a summary of the most common indications for pediatric spinal MR Imaging.

In conclusion, all the authors involved in this review have made efforts to produce articles that it is hoped offer a helpful overview of the main topics about spinal pathologies a radiologist may encounter during his professional career.

Mario Muto, MD
Neuroradiology Department
Cardarelli Hospital
Via Petrarca 57
Naples 80100, Italy

E-mail address:
mutomar@tiscali.it

Neuroimaging of Spinal Instability

Mario Muto, MD[a],*, Francesco Giurazza, MD[b], Gianluigi Guarnieri, MD[a], Roberto Izzo, MD[a], Alvaro Diano, MD[a]

KEYWORDS

- Back pain • Spinal instability • Dynamic radiography • CT • Dynamic MRI • Open MRI scanner

KEY POINTS

- Degenerative, traumatic, and neoplastic instabilities are based on different pathophysiologic mechanisms, so each pattern requires a peculiar integrated clinical-radiologic approach.
- Dynamic radiographs with upright true lateral neutral-flexion-extension projections are still the most widely used imaging approach to diagnose instability in the daily practice.
- In traumatic instability, computerized tomography (CT) is the preferred image modality because it is able to detect quickly even the tiniest unstable fractures with reduced patient manipulation.
- Conventional MRI acquired in supine rest position often correlates poorly with clinical findings because of the loaded positional dependence of patient symptoms.
- Novel dynamic MRI approaches simulate closely the pathologic conditions that elicit symptoms in patients with instability, providing strict linkage between clinical status and imaging.

INTRODUCTION

The human spine is a complex biomechanical system composed of multiple articular structures controlled by muscles. It has 2 principal crucial functions: support and protection. The spine supports the head and trunk and protects the spinal cord, nerve roots, and vertebral arteries during every movement. Furthermore, it transfers power forces between upper and lower limbs.

These functions presuppose spine stability; however, even though several articles have been published about this concept, a consensus definition of stability is still lacking.

Clinical problems of the human spine continue to be prevalent in society. Examples include low back pain, sciatica, spinal deformity in both adults and children, spinal tumors, and spinal injury, including trauma to the spinal cord.[1] Frequently these are related with a loss of stability (instability) particularly at the lumbar level. Traumatic, neoplastic, and degenerative instability are important causes of spinal pain and disability.[2]

Conventional radiology with dynamic projections has long been considered the technical reference to assess the degree of instability,[3] and different methods have been developed to assess the presence of listhesis; however, radiography has proved inadequate to assess stability in case of spinal fractures.[4] Furthermore, because patients with instability frequently present concomitant disk and radicular pathologies, conventional radiography is limited by its diagnostic use in the assessment of these structures. CT, instead, yields high-resolution reconstructions in every spatial plane to detect even the tiniest fractures, revealing potentially unstable lesions.

MRI is the only imaging modality that directly assesses ligaments integrity, which is crucial for spine stability. In the past 2 decades, novel loaded

The authors have nothing to disclose.
a Neuroradiology Department, Cardarelli Hospital, Via Cardarelli 9, Naples 80131, Italy; b Radiology Department, Università Campus Bio-Medico di Roma, Via Alvaro del Portillo 200, Rome 00100, Italy
* Corresponding author.
E-mail address: mutomar@tiscali.it

mri.theclinics.com

MRI systems have been developed to evaluate instability in a more realistic pathologic condition, adding relevant information to conventional supine MRI.[5–7]

This article reviews the basic pathologic concepts of spinal instability and describes the role of the different imaging techniques in the assessment of this clinical issue.

PATHOLOGIC PRINCIPLES OF INSTABILITY

Spinal stability depends on the interaction of 2 strictly related elements, column and muscles, under the control of the central nervous system.[8] The loss of stability leads to instability, because for stability, a univocal definition has not been agreed on, even if it remains critical in the surgical decision-making process. White and Panjabi[9] defined instability as "the loss of the ability of the spine under physiologic loads to maintain its patterns of displacement so there is no initial or additional neurologic deficit, no major deformity, and no incapacitating pain."[9] Pope and colleagues[10] intended instability as a loss of stiffness leading to abnormal and increased movement in the motion segments. Spinal movements are 3-D with coupled movements, so spine instability always causes dysfunctional motions in more than 1 direction.

There are different patterns of instability based on the pathophysiologic mechanisms that sustain the process: degenerative, traumatic, and neoplastic.

Degenerative Instability

Spinal degenerative instability is a common cause of pain and disability. This pathologic process starts with the lesion of a component of the column, leading to an inappropriate response of the muscles and consequently an erroneous positional feedback of the column. In this way, a vicious circle causes a chronic dysfunction and pain through 3 steps, the degenerative cascade: dysfunction, instability, and restabilization.

Dysfunction phase

The dysfunction phase is characterized by an occasional undefined low back pain, with no or minimal changes in the spinal joints; frequently in this situation no imaging findings are appreciable.

Instability phase

In the instability phase, back pain becomes more and more frequent to chronic. Multiple signs are appreciable on radiologic examinations (x-ray, MRI, and CT scans), such as facets degeneration and disk space narrowing. These elements lead to abnormal vertebral movement and alignment,

up to anterolisthesis or retrolisthesis. At the beginning of the instability phase, the process is usually limited to a single joint but then, it involves the adjacent joints, resulting in a multifocal pathology. End plate, peduncle, and isthmic edema; Modic changes; traction spurs; extended discal vacuum; facets gapping with joint effusion or vacuum; synovial cysts; annular tears; spondylolysthesis; and retrolysthesis are typical imaging findings of the full-blown disease.[2] Sometimes on standard supine scans, signs of instability are available but vertebral alignment is preserved; however, this alignment is a misleading condition due to the absence of load bearing. In these cases, a dynamic radiograph or an upright MRI is suitable to diagnose occult instability.[11]

Restabilization phase

In the final phase, restabilization, structural compensatory remodeling phenomena bring reduced mobility and stiffness. Marginal osteophytes; disk collapse; radial expansion of vertebral bodies and facets; and end plate, spinous, and transverse sclerosis: all these remodeling processes interrupt vertebral slippage but also block physiologic movements.

Traumatic Instability

Unlike degenerative instability, the relationship between imaging findings and clinical symptoms tends to be more direct in traumatic spinal instability. Every time a trauma damages a column element, it produces a certain degree of instability; all spinal components contribute to stability. Different studies have analyzed the effects of trauma on the spine and different models have been developed. Denis[12] proposed a model formed by 3 vertical columns: an anterior column, including the anterior halves of the bodies and disks with the adjacent anterior longitudinal ligament; a middle column, including the posterior half of the bodies and disks with posterior longitudinal ligament; and a posterior column, consisting of neural arches and the posterior ligamentous complex, including the supraspinous, interspinous, and flava ligaments and facet joint capsules. Denis assessed that instability was due to the simultaneous failure of at least 2 columns, creating situations of instability.[12] Today Denis's model remains among the most accepted references.

Although a considerable amount of energy is required to produce the first injury in a vertebra, just a small additional trauma is sufficient to convert a lesion from stable to unstable and to switch from conservative treatment to surgical stabilization.[2]

The thoracolumbar spine is the most common site afflicted by trauma; L1 is the most common vertebra followed by T12.[13] Its predilection and vulnerability for injury stems from the following reasons: (1) mobility: the thoracolumbar spine presents a high degree of mobility, so is subjected to all kinds of forces, resulting in a district highly vulnerable to fractures; (2) transition zone: the thoracolumbar region is relatively straight (kyphosis from 0°–10°) and situated between the kyphotic thoracic and lordotic lumbar spine; unlike the thoracic spine, the absence of costovertebral structures no longer protects the thoracolumbar zone; and (3) facet joints: facet joints of the thoracic spine are coronally oriented to resist flexion-extension and that of lumbar spine are sagittally oriented to allow flexion-extension. In the thoracolumbar area, facet joints show a transition from predominantly coronal to predominantly sagittal orientation.[13]

Thoracolumbar fractures have been classified by Magerl and colleagues[14] into 3 main groups: A, B, and C types (each 1 divided into 3 subgroups), corresponding to increasing degrees of instability; this classification system is based on progressive morphologic damage determined by 3 fundamental forces: compression, distraction, and axial torque (rotation). Type A injuries are either stable or partially compromised but never completely unstable, because the posterior longitudinal ligament is intact, while the degree of stability progresses from the most stable type A to the most unstable type A3; types B1 and B2 are unstable in flexion because of the posterior ligament injury while stability in the extension is maintained by an intact anterior ligament; type B3 injuries are unstable in extension but may be stable in flexion, if the posterior ligament is intact; and all type C injuries are unstable.

The most important finding in recognizing stable versus unstable fractures is the state of the posterior ligaments; the status of posterior ligaments after an injury is of great importance for the stability of the injured spine. In burst fractures, the condition of the posterior column suggests fracture instability, which increases remarkably in cases of lesions to the posterior ligaments.[2]

MRI is the only imaging modality able to assess changes in ligaments with significant accuracy and has a crucial role in treatment choice. MRI interpretation in this clinical scenario, however, needs to be improved. It does not find clear signs of ligament discontinuity but just signal modifications occurring in and around apparently continuous ligaments: the clinical meaning of these findings is still unclear. On the other hand, a ligament must not necessarily be torn to become biomechanically ineffective, and the absence of signal modifications cannot always exclude instability.[15]

Neoplastic Instability

Spinal instability as a result of a neoplastic process differs significantly from high-energy traumatic injuries in the pattern of bony and ligamentous involvement, potential for healing, neurologic manifestations, and bone quality. It requires a specific and different set of criteria for stability assessment.

Neoplastic spine instability has been defined by the Spine Oncology Study Group as loss of spinal integrity as a result of a neoplastic process associated with movement-related pain, symptomatic or progressive deformity, and/or neural compromise under physiologic loads.[16]

Spinal Instability Neoplastic Score

A panel of expert members from Spine Oncology Study Group developed the Spinal Instability Neoplastic Score, taking into account 6 components, each receiving a score that rises based on the rate of instability. The minimum score is 0 and maximum is 18. Scores of 0 to 6 denote stability, scores of 7 to 12 denote indeterminate (possibly impending) instability, and scores of 13 to 18 denote instability. Patients with Spinal Instability Neoplastic Score scores of 7 to 18 warrant surgical consultation. The 6 components are spine location, mechanical pain, bone lesion quality, spinal alignment, vertebral body collapse, and posterolateral involvement of spinal elements.

Impending spinal instability affects clinical decision making in oncologic spinal disease. In patients with neoplastic spinal disease without neurologic deficit, it is crucial to recognize which situations are unstable or may lead to spinal instability and neurologic injury. This allows proper stabilization of patients with severe mechanical pain and hopefully prevents painful collapse with neurologic consequences.

IMAGING IN SPINAL INSTABILITY

Various techniques have been developed over the past decades to evaluate the presence of spinal instability both clinically and radiologically. The most widely used approach is lumbar flexion-extension radiography but CT and MRI are also applied in this field with dedicated protocol.

Dynamic Radiography

Radiographs are acquired in dynamic modality with upright anterior-posterior and true lateral neutral-flexion-extension projections[17] (**Fig. 1**).

The degree of listhesis is usually measured according to the method described by White and

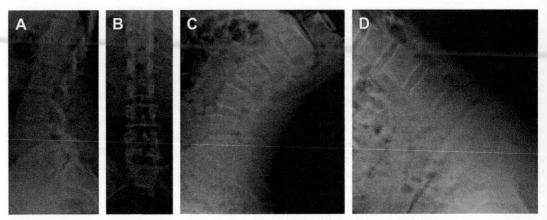

Fig. 1. Standard projections of a dynamic lumbar radiography with (*A, C, D*) upright neutral-flexion-extension lateral projections and (*B*) upright anteroposterior projection. A low-grade L4-L5 anterolisthesis is appreciable in the neutral lateral projection that, however, is not further evident in flexion-extension.

Panjabi[18] or by applying the measurement method proposed by Dupuis and colleagues.[19] In the first case, a baseline is drawn along the upper end plate of the vertebral body while 2 other perpendicular lines are drawn passing through the superior posterior edge of the vertebral body and the posterior inferior edge of the adjacent vertebral body; the distance between the 2 perpendicular lines represents the degree of listhesis and is significant if more than 3 mm. In the second approach, the listhesis is evaluated as the slip percentage, considered the ratio between the sagittal translational displacement and the vertebral body depth, and significant if exceeding 8% (L1-L5) or 9% (L5-S1).[17,19]

No definite agreement on the optimum approach to evaluate segmental instability has been reached, however, and there have been studies calling for reproducibility of such images; flexion-extension radiographs in the standing position are dependent on patient cooperation, which has challenged the relevance of such images in the evaluation of vertebral instability in the view of some investigators.[20–22]

Recently, Pieper and colleagues[17] have attempted to evaluate if it is necessary to acquire both positions, extension and flexion radiographs, in addition to neutral standing images; they concluded that extension views could be omitted in a routine work-up for the evaluation of ventral instability in spondylolisthesis, because they do not add relevant information—nothing differing from that in the neutral standing position—and to keep the radiation dose as low as reasonably achievable.

Computerized Tomography

Conventional radiology is inadequate for the assessment of stability in case of trauma; it has

been proved to miss 61% of all cervical fractures[3] and flexion-extension radiographies are considered to add little or nothing in the assessment of cervical unstable lesions.[23] On the other hand, CT can detect even the tiniest fractures in the middle and posterior columns, revealing potentially unstable lesions, and also allows an excellent evaluation of vertebral alignment and the spatial position of dislocated bone fragments (**Fig. 2**). Hogan and colleagues[24] found a negative predictive value for CT of 98.9% for ligamentous lesions and 100% predictive value for unstable cervical spine injuries, concluding that a normal CT study alone may exclude unstable cervical injuries.

As in the cervical district, in a comparative study of detecting thoracolumbar fractures, the sensitivity of CT reached 97.2%,[25] whereas up to two-thirds of all unstable fractures were missed by conventional radiographs.

CT can yield high-resolution reformatting in every spatial plane, starting from isotropic image voxels, to detect even the tiniest fractures in the middle and posterior columns, revealing potentially unstable lesions.[26] CT also allows an excellent evaluation of vertebral alignment and the spatial position of dislocated bone fragments, both in the cervical and thoracolumbar districts when conventional radiography failed.[2] It must also be considered that thanks to the greater accuracy, high speed, and reduced patient manipulation, CT is the preferred imaging modality in acute multitrauma patients.

In degenerative instability, CT could provide indirect signs of instability and relevant information about predisposing anatomic factors, such as facet joint asymmetry, unilateral recess stenosis, and foraminal disk herniation, that may lead to an abnormal axial rotation of a vertebra on the

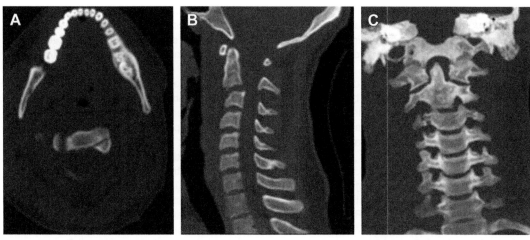

Fig. 2. CT of a 23-year-old man crushed with motorbike. (*A*) Axial CT demonstrated the fracture of the postero-lateral left portion of the body of C2; (*B*) sagittal lateral reconstruction demonstrated the fracture of the anterior portion of the upper lamina of C3 and C2-C3 anterolisthesis; and (*C*) coronal volume rendering reconstruction revealed a right lateral subluxation of C2-C3.

subjacent one; these findings finally could be responsible of rotational listhesis.[27]

Axial Load Computerized Tomography

Some investigators[28,29] proposed CT for studying spine sagittal alignment during axial load to simulate the standing loading posture. Dedicated compression devices have been developed to expose lumbar spine to an axial force similar to that in the spine in the standing position; the value of this force in normal conditions is approximately 50% of body weight.[30] Hioki and colleagues[28] enrolled a small population (14 healthy young subjects) and performed supine CT scans (slice thickness: 3 mm) positioning a compression device (DynaWell; DynaWell, Las Vegas, Nevada) consisting of a foot plate, a shoulder harness, and interconnecting straps; the amount of compression was adjustable and measured by force transducers in the foot plate; in this study, patients rested in the supine position on a stretcher for 1 hour and then they were placed on the CT table in a relaxed supine position with the hips and knees straight and extended. CT of the lumbar spine was performed first without applying any axial compression force and then after axial compression for 5 minutes. Analyzing the images after reconstruction in sagittal planes obtained at the midline of the lumbar spine, the authors concluded that the compression device simulated the lumbar segmental alignment change from supine to standing posture in L1/2, L2/3, L3/4, and L4/5; however, in L5/S1, axial loading using the DynaWell altered lumbar segmental alignment

with a kyphotic change. Compared with other modern techniques, this approach, although having economical advantages, presented some relevant limitations because the compression devices do not completely simulate the condition of the lumbar spine in the standing position and do not allow an accurate evaluation the spinal canal; finally, it must also be taken into account that other approaches, such as dynamic MRI, are free from radiation exposure.

Axial Load MR Imaging

Until a few years ago, radiograph was the only practicable imaging modality for the spine in the upright position. This examination is valid and useful for evaluating spinal curvatures, but it shows its limitations when the assessment should be directed to disk structures or when it is necessary to obtain measurements free from problems due to overlapping of anatomic images.[31]

A first attempt to evaluate the spine under the loading condition was done with the axial load technique both with CT (discussed previously) and MRI, which simulates physiologic loading of the spine in the orthostatic position.

MRI is a noninvasive diagnostic tool that is widely used to evaluate various diseases of the lumbar spine. Because the conventional MRI examinations of the spine usually are performed in supine position, in functional rest, the loading conditions differ from those known to elicit the symptoms in patients affected by lumbar spine instability; this is frequently exacerbated by upright standing and hidden in the supine position.[5,32]

In supine position, various pathologic features, including deformation of the dural sac, nerve roots compression, the presence of bulging disk, thickening of the ligamentum flavum, and/or narrowing of the intervertebral foramen, can remain undetected compared with that observed in the standing position.[33] Therefore, it should be considered that pathologic findings could be invisible in images obtained with the conventional supine position, so a certain rate of false-negative results in MRI should be taken into account.

As for axial load CT (discussed previously), a compression device for performing axial loading of the lumbar spine with the patient in the supine position has been developed for MRI[34,35] to simulate a physiologic normal weight-bearing condition in the upright position. Sagittal T2-weighted turbo spin-echo sequences are acquired with a spine array coil (slice thickness: 4 mm) and images are evaluated at the midline of the lumbar spine.

Kanno and colleagues[32] demonstrated that axial-loaded MRI more accurately estimates the degree of listhesis in the standing position than conventional MRI, with the degree of listhesis on axial-loaded MRI significantly more correlated with that observed on sagittal x-ray studies in the upright position.

Although results were certainly interesting and allowed better assessment in relation to the higher signal-to-noise ratio afforded by the high-field equipment, the technique has not achieved a general consensus.

Studies[28,36] have demonstrated that the parameters of the alignment of the lumbar spine under axial loading in the supine position, including the intervertebral angle, disk height, and lordotic angle, are not perfectly equal to those observed in the actual standing position and that the degree of axial loading to the lumbar spine in the standing position is not correctly replicated when a patient is in the supine position; these differences in spinal alignment may result in a discrepancy in the degree of listhesis between that measured on radiograph studies in the standing position and that observed on axial-loaded MRI. The degree of listhesis on axial-loaded MRI is significantly correlated with, but not completely equal to, that observed on x-ray images. This issue is related to a relevant flaw of the axial-loaded MRI: this approach does not consider the influence that head/body weight and muscle activation have on the lumbar spine stability.[7,37,38]

Dynamic MR Imaging

At the end of 1990s, the first studies were published[6,38] about dynamic MRI using an open magnet that allowed upright scanning in either seated or standing body position. The reported results were not convincing, however, with limited information gained in addition to that from standard MRI.[27]

Currently, the technological advancement of open MRI scanners allows better performance in terms of assessment of spinal instability and variations of some pathologic conditions from recumbent to upright position (**Fig. 3**). These devices also have the advantage of eliminating a patient's feeling of claustrophobia, which sometimes limits diagnostic evaluation of the spine.[39–42]

Usually the magnetic fields are 0.25 T, 0.5 T, and 0.6 T. Images are obtained with patient both supine and upright in the flexed, extended, rotated, standing, and bending positions.[3] The standard protocol usually include the following sequences acquired with dedicated surface coils:

- Supine: sagittal T1-weighted spin-echo, sagittal and axial T2-weighted turbo spin-echo with and without fat saturation
- Upright (after repetition of the positioning scout): sagittal and axial T2-weighted turbo spin-echo

The slice thickness is 3.5 mm to 4.5 mm with a gap of 0.5 mm.

Apart from instability assessment, in many cases dynamic MRI has proved[3,5,43–45] to reveal disk-radicular conflicts not depicted on conventional MRI studies (**Figs. 4** and **5**).

Splendiani and colleagues[5] found in a large sample of patients significant differences in the evaluation of degenerative aspects analyzed with dynamic MRI in the transition from standing to supine position; in particular, they reported a significant number of positive cases (715 of 1178 patients; $P = .0004$) with translational intervertebral movements greater than 3 mm and new appearance of spondylolisthesis in 9.5% of the cases. Furthermore, with the passage from supine to upright position, the appearance of disk protrusions was significantly detected in 11% of the cases as well as the increase or appearance of spinal canal stenosis in 9.2% of the cases; these data are in agreement with other previous published studies[43–45] performed with open dynamic MRI magnet on smaller sample.

In another study on a sample of 57 symptomatic subjects for low back pain, Tarantino and colleagues[31] reported that 70% of patients, on visual qualitative analysis only, had an increment of disk protrusions and/or spondylolisthesis found in the upright position and in 3 cases, in the upright position only, an interarticular pseudocyst was found.

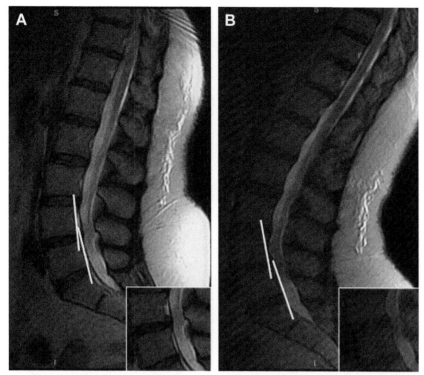

Fig. 3. Dynamic MRI of a 53-year-old man affected by lumbar pain acquired on a 0.5-T magnet. T2-weighted turbo spin-echo sequence in sagittal midline in (A) supine and (B) upright standing. L4-L5 anterolisthesis becomes evident in upright (squared enlargements). White lines indicate the posterior walls alignment.

In the degenerative instability process, the restabilization phase is challenging to interpret without the aid of a dynamic study of the spine: it concerns both the nerve root compression at the level of foramina, due to osteophytes, and the activation of postural effects of body weight mediated by abdominal and paraspinal muscles, moving from orthostatic to standing position.

Some investigators[3,45] also underlined the more significant clinical meaning of imaging findings, concluding that dynamic MRI offered an optimal linkage of the patient's syndrome with the imaging

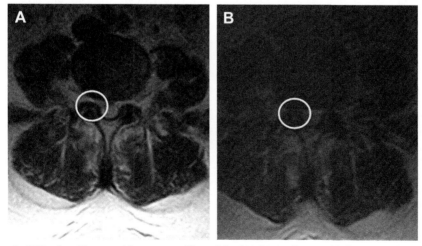

Fig. 4. Dynamic MRI of a 61-year-old woman affected by lumbar pain acquired on a 0.5-T magnet. Axial T2-weighted turbo spin-echo sequence in (A) supine and (B) upright standing. Right discal protrusion with intra-foraminal radicular conflict (white circle) becomes evident in upright.

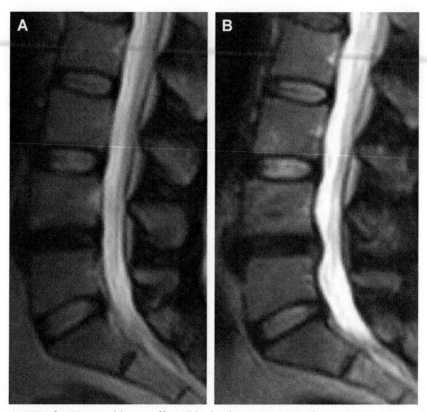

Fig. 5. Dynamic MRI of a 56-year-old man affected by lumbar pain acquired on a 0.25-T magnet. T2-weighted turbo spin-echo sequence in sagittal midline in (*A*) supine and (*B*) upright standing. L4-L5 discal protrusion becomes evident in upright; the disk appears clearly dehydrated (*dark disk sign*).

abnormalities responsible for the clinical presentation, thereby allowing for the first time an improvement at once in both imaging sensitivity and specificity.

Because of the relative novelty of this approach, clinical and diagnostic criteria have not yet been clearly defined, so further clinical trials are required.

LIMITATIONS

Dynamic MRI is a promising technique but entails some limitations,[3,5,27,29,31,45] first of all represented by the low-field magnet resulting in a low signal-to-noise ratio and an overall reduced image quality compared with the common high-field magnet. Another important limit is the long scanning time compared with conventional supine MRI because of the additional acquisitions in upright standing; apart from creating possible management inconveniences in the daily session, this issue can produce pain problems and motion artifacts because symptomatic patients may find it difficult to maintain the immobility necessary for the whole duration of the imaging acquisition in

the upright position.[31] Consequently, difficulties can occur in reproducing the positioning between the sequences. These limits could be partially balanced by the use of 3-D scan protocol with a precise postprocessing reconstruction using the MPR algorithm with an effective thickness of 1 mm, parallel to the vertebral end plate in the coronal and sagittal planes.[44] Finally, some investigators also reported an occasional difficulty encountered in evaluating the most lateral areas of the spine, such as exit foramen and lateral recesses,[6,31] due to section thickness and degree of patient rotation and lateral flexion.

SUMMARY

The spine is a complex structure, the integrity of which depends on multiple anatomic elements that are functionally strictly related to each other. Different pathologic processes can modify this biomechanical balance, creating spinal instability and consequent back pain and functional impairment.

Multiple imaging modalities are used in daily practice to assess this clinical condition; however, because of the lack of a univocal definition of instability, the diagnosis is not always correctly obtained. Nowadays novel MRI systems allow studying the spine in more realistic loading conditions able to elicit symptoms in patients affected by spine instability. Further trials are required to clearly understand the correct diagnostic pathway in the light of these new technologies to choose the best therapeutic approach.

REFERENCES

1. Oxland TR. Fundamental biomechanics of the spine—What we have learned in the past 25 years and future directions. J Biomech 2015. http://dx.doi.org/10.1016/j.jbiomech.2015.10.035.
2. Izzo R, Guarnieri G, Guglielmi G, et al. Biomechanics of the spine. Part II: Spinal instability. Eur J Radiol 2013;1:127–38.
3. Alyas F, Connell D, Saifuddin A. Upright positional MRI of the lumbar spine. Clin Radiol 2008;63: 1035–48.
4. Poonnoose PM, Ravichandran G, McClelland MR. Missed and mismanaged injuries of the spinal cord. J Trauma 2002;53:314–20.
5. Splendiani A, Perri M, Grattacaso G, et al. Magnetic resonance imaging (MRI) of the lumbar spine with dedicated G-scan machine in the upright position: a retrospective study and our experience in 10 years with 4305 patients. Radiol Med 2016;121(1): 38–44.
6. Weishaupt D, Schmid MR, Zanetti M, et al. Positional MR imaging of the lumbar spine: does it demonstrate nerve root compromise not visible at conventional MR imaging? Radiology 2000;215:247–53.
7. Manenti G, Liccardo G, Sergiacomi G, et al. Axial loading MRI of the lumbar spine. In Vivo 2003;17: 413–20.
8. Izzo R, Guarnieri G, Guglielmi G, et al. Biomechanics of the spine. Part I: Spinal stability. Eur J Radiol 2013;(1):118–26.
9. White AA III, Panjabi MM. The basic kinematics of the human spine. Spine 1978;3(1):12–20.
10. Pope MH, Panjabi M. Biomechanical definitions of spinal instability. Spine 1985;10:255–6.
11. Izzo R, Popolizio T, D'Aprile P, et al. Spinal pain. Eur J Radiol 2015;84:746–56.
12. Denis F. The three columns spine and its significance in the classification of acute thoracolumbar spinal injuries. Spine 1983;8:817–31.
13. Azam Q, Sadat-Ali M. The concept of evolution of thoracolumbar fracture classifications helps in surgical decisions. Asian Spine J 2015;9(6):984–94.
14. Magerl F, Aebi M, Gertzbein SD, et al. A comprehensive classification of thoracic and lumbar injuries. Eur Spine J 1994;3:184–201.
15. Lee HM, Kim HS, Kim DJ, et al. Reliability of magnetic resonance imaging in detecting posterior ligament complex injury in thoracolumbar spinal fractures. Spine 2000;15(2516):2079–84.
16. Fisher CG, Di Paola CP, Ryken TC, et al. A novel classification system for spinal instability in neoplastic disease. an evidence-based approach and expert consensus from the Spine Oncology Study Group. Spine 2010;35(22):E1221–9.
17. Pieper CC, Groetz SF, Nadal J, et al. Radiographic evaluation of ventral instability in lumbar spondylolisthesis: do we need extension radiographs in routine exams? Eur Spine J 2014;23:96–101.
18. White A, Panjabi M. Clinical biomechanics of the spine. 2nd edition. Philadelphia: Lippincott; 1990.
19. Dupuis PR, Yong-Hing K, Cassidy JD, et al. Radiological diagnosis of degenerative lumbar spinal instability. Spine 1985;10:262–6.
20. Nizard RS, Wybler M, Laredo JD. Radiologic assessment of lumbar intervertebral instability and degenerative spondylolisthesis. Radiol Clin North Am 2001;39:55–71.
21. Dvorak J, Panjabi MM, Chang D, et al. Functional radiographic diagnosis of the lumbar spine: flexion- extension and lateral bending. Spine 1991;16:562–71.
22. Posner I, White AA 3rd, Edwards WT, et al. A biomechanical analysis of the clinical stability of the lumbar and lumbosacral spine. Spine 1982;7: 374–89.
23. Knopp R, Parker J, Tashjian J, et al. Defining radiographic criteria for flexion–extension studies of the cervical spine. Ann Emerg Med 2001;38(1):31–5.
24. Hogan GJ, Mirvis SE, Shanmuganathan K, et al. Exclusion of unstable cervical spine injury in obtunded patients with blunt trauma: is MR imaging needed when multi-detector row CT findings are normal? Radiology 2005;237:106–13.
25. Wintermark M, Mouhsine E, Theurmann N, et al. Thoracolumbar spine fractures in patients who have sustained severe trauma: depiction with multi-detector row CT. Radiology 2003;227:681–9.
26. Campbell SE, Phillips CD, Dubovsky E, et al. The value of CT in determining potential instability of simple wedge-compression fractures of the lumbar spine. AJNR Am J Neuroradiol 1995;16:1385–92.
27. Leone A, Guglielmi G, Cassar-Pullicino VN, et al. Lumbar intervertebral instability: a review. Radiology 2007;245:62–77.
28. Hioki A, Miyamoto K, Sakai H, et al. Lumbar axial loading device alters lumbar sagittal alignment differently from upright stand- ing position: a computed tomography study. Spine 2010;35: 995–1001.
29. Willen J, Danielson B. The diagnostic effect from axial loading of the lumbar spine during computed tomography and magnetic resonance imaging in

patients with degenerative disorders. Spine 2001; 26:2607–14.

30. Reynolds HM. The Inertial proportion of the body and its segments. In: Staff of the Anthropology Research Project, Webb Associates, editor. NASA reference publication no. 1024. anthropomtric source book: vol. I. Anthropometry for designers. (OH): Yellow Springs; 1978. p. 4.31–9.

31. Tarantino U, Fanucci E, Iundusi R, et al. Lumbar spine MRI in upright position for diagnosing acute and chronic low back pain: statistical analysis of morphological changes. J Orthop Traumatol 2013; 14:15–22.

32. Kanno H, Ozawa H, Koizumi Y, et al. Changes in lumbar spondylolisthesis on axial-loaded MRI: do they reproduce the positional changes in the degree of olisthesis observed on X-ray images in the standing position? Spine J 2015;15:1255–62.

33. Kanno H, Endo T, Ozawa H, et al. Axial loading during magnetic resonance imaging in patients with lumbar spinal canal stenosis: does it reproduce the positional change of the dural sac detected by upright myelography? Spine 2012;37:E985–92.

34. Danielson BI, Willen J, Gaulitz A, et al. Axial loading of the spine during CT and MR in patients with suspected lumbar spinal stenosis. Acta Radiol 1998;39: 604–11.

35. Willen J, Danielson B, Gaulitz A, et al. Dynamic effects on the lumbar spinal canal: axially loaded CT-myelography and MRI in patients with sciatica and/or neurogenic claudication. Spine 1997;22:2968–76.

36. Wessberg P, Danielson BI, Willen J. Comparison of Cobb angles in idiopathic scoliosis on standing radiographs and supine axially loaded MRI. Spine 2006;31:3039–44.

37. Vitzthum HE, Konig A, Seifert V. Dynamic examination of the lumbar spine by using vertical, open magnetic resonance imaging. J Neurosurg 2000; 93:58–64.

38. Wildermuth S, Zanetti M, Duewell S, et al. Lumbar spine: quantitative and qualitative assessment of positional (upright flexion and extension) MR imaging and myelography. Radiology 1998;207:391–8.

39. Madsen R, Jensen TS, Pope M, et al. The effect of body position and axial load on spinal canal morphology: an MRI study of central spinal stenosis. Spine (Phila Pa 1976) 2008;33:61–7.

40. Danielson B, Willen J. Axially loaded magnetic resonance image of the lumbar spine in asymptomatic individuals. Spine (Phila Pa 1976) 2001;26:2601–6.

41. Schmid MR, Stucki G, Duewell S, et al. Changes in cross-sectional measurements of the spinal canal and intervertebral foramina as a function of body position: in vivo studies on an open-configuration MR system. AJR Am J Roentgenol 1999;172:1095–102.

42. Vitaz TW, Shields CB, Raque GH, et al. Dynamic weight-bearing cervical magnetic resonance imaging: technical review and preliminary results. South Med J 2004;97:456–61.

43. McGregor AH, Anderton L, Gedroyc WM, et al. The use of interventional open MRI to assess the kinematics of the lumbar spine in patients with spondylolisthesis. Spine 2002;27:1582–6.

44. Splendiani A, Ferrari F, Barile A, et al. Occult neural foraminal stenosis caused by association between disc degeneration and facet joint osteoarthritis: demonstration with dedicated upright MRI system. Radiol Med 2014;119(3):164–74.

45. Jinkins JR, Dworkin JS, Damadian RV. Upright, weight-bearing, dynamic-kinetic MRI of the spine: initial results. Eur Radiol 2005;15(9):1815–25.

The Degenerative Spine

Frédéric Clarençon, MD, PhD[a,b,*], Bruno Law-Ye, MD[b,c],
Peggy Bienvenot, MD[c], Évelyne Cormier, MD[a], Jacques Chiras, MD[a,b]

KEYWORDS

• Spine • MR imaging • Degenerative • Arthrosis • Intervertebral disc • Herniation • Modic

KEY POINTS

- MR imaging has a key role for exploration of spine degenerative disease.
- Intervertebral disc fissures are optimally depicted on T2-weighted imaging.
- Spine MR imaging should systematically be performed for cases of back pain associated with neurologic deficit.
- MR imaging is the best imaging modality for the exploration of spinal canal stenosis.

INTRODUCTION

Degenerative disease of the spine is a leading cause of back pain and radiculopathy, and a frequent indication for spine MR imaging.[1] Disc degeneration, disc protrusion/herniation, discarthrosis, spinal canal stenosis, facet joint arthrosis as well as interspinous processes arthrosis may require an MR imaging workup. This review presents the MR imaging patterns of these diseases and describes the benefits of the MR imaging in these indications compared with the other imaging modalities like plain radiographs or computed tomography (CT) scan.

INDICATIONS FOR SPINE MR IMAGING/ IMAGING PROTOCOLS

In most cases, back pain does not require imaging if no neurologic deficit is observed on clinical examination. However, when pain lasts for more than 4 weeks despite analgesic medications, imaging of the spine is required. The first line imaging technique is the conventional spine radiograph or spine CT scan, except in case of neurologic deficit.

In some cases, spine MR imaging should, however, be performed:

- Low back pain complicated by radiculopathy (cruralgia, sciatica);
- Symptoms related to spinal canal stenosis;
- Radiculopathy with neurologic deficit; and
- Cauda equina syndrome.

Compared with conventional radiographs, MR imaging of the spine offers the possibility to directly visualize the intervertebral disc, as well as the nerve roots and the spinal cord.

Compared with spine CT scan, MR imaging of the spine has the advantage of being a nonirradiant examination. Additionally, it helps to see the spinal cord clearly and may help to distinguish recurrent disc protrusion versus fibrosis in a postoperative condition or to detect an inflammatory lesion or tumor disease.[2] The major limitation of this imaging modality is that the acquisition may be long and may be hampered by motion artifacts, especially in patients who are in a good deal of pain. CT of the spine presents some other advantages compared with MR imaging, like better visualization of osteophytes, intradiscal gas (vacuum disc), and calcifications.

It is accepted commonly that a MR imaging protocol of the spine should contain at least 2 orthogonal plans. The surface coils are the most

The authors have nothing to disclose.

[a] Department of Interventional Neuroradiology, Pitié-Salpêtrière Hospital, 47, Bd de l'Hôpital, Paris 75013, France; [b] Paris VI University, Pierre et Marie Curie, 47, Bd de l'Hôpital, Paris 75013, France; [c] Department of Diagnostic and Functional Neuroradiology, Pitié-Salpêtrière Hospital, 47, Bd de l'Hôpital, Paris 75013, France
* Corresponding author. Service de Neuroradiologie, Pitié-Salpêtrière Hospital, 47, Bd de l'Hôpital, Paris 75013, France.
E-mail address: fredclare5@msn.com

Magn Reson Imaging Clin N Am 24 (2016) 495–513
http://dx.doi.org/10.1016/j.mric.2016.04.008

commonly used. The most widely used protocol for exploration of degenerative disease of the spine includes: sagittal T1 and T2 weighted images (WI) and sagittal (or coronal) short tau inversion recovery (STIR)-WI. The latter sequence helps in the characterization of edema of the medullary bone.[3] Axial T2-WI acquisitions are systematically performed on the 3 to 4 last lumbar disc levels to depict potential foraminal or extraforminal disc herniation. Axial T2-WI also helps to pinpoint the precise relationship between the disc bulging/herniation and the surrounding nervous structures (nerve roots and spinal cord). For cervical spine exploration, a 3-dimensional gradient echo sequence provides a slice thickness of less than 1 mm, helping to see more precisely the intervertebral foramina and the nerve roots. CUBE T2 acquisition may also be valuable because it allows for multiplanar reconstructions, offering a better visualization of nerve roots compression. Finally, contrast media injection should only be performed postoperatively to distinguish recurrent herniation from fibrosis[2] or to help in distinguishing a disc-free fragment from a nerve root tumor.[4] The whole spinal cord should be explored by the MR imaging acquisition when neurologic symptoms related to spinal cord compression are observed on clinical evaluation. Indeed, compressive disc herniation may be multifocal.[5]

DISC DEGENERATION

The intervertebral discs are located between the endplates of adjacent vertebral bodies; they have a cushion shape and allow the mobility of one vertebral body over another. They are cartilaginous structures; their composition is divided into the nucleus pulposus in the central aspect of the disc and the annulus fibrosus at the peripheral aspect. The annulus fibrosus and the nucleus pulposus are both made of collagen (type II for the nucleus pulposus and type I for the annulus fibrosus) and proteoglycans.[6] The nucleus pulposus is made of more than 80% of water and has a gelatinous texture. The annulus fibrosus consists of concentric rings or lamellae, with fibers in the outer lamellae continuing into the longitudinal ligaments and vertebral bodies. The collagen lamellae are denser at the peripheral aspect of the annulus. The Sharpey fibers are dense collagen fibers located on outer aspect of the annulus that attach the intervertebral disc to the adjacent endplates.[6–9] The intervertebral disc is also attached ventrally and dorsally to the anterior and posterior longitudinal ligaments (PLL), respectively.

Disc changes may be related to aging or to degeneration if repeated, clinically significant

mechanical constraints are exerted on the intervertebral disc. With aging, disc cells biological changes are observed, mainly cell type alteration within the nucleus pulposus, cell death, and alteration of cell phenotype compromising their ability to synthetize normal matrix components.[10] Additionally, increased inflammatory response and enhanced catabolic metabolism leading to breakdown of the extracellular matrix are observed in the degenerated disc.[11]

The term "disc degeneration" include the following pathomechanisms and imaging patterns: desiccation, disc space narrowing, disc bulging, disc herniation, disc tears or fissures, intradiscal gas, disc calcification, inflammatory/sclerotic changes of the vertebral endplates, and marginal osteophytes.

Progressive loss of disc water is called "desiccation" and appears on T2-WI imaging as a more or less marked reduction of the normal hyperintense signal within the intervertebral disc.[12] This decrease in signal intensity on T2-WI is thus an early surrogate marker of intervertebral disc degeneration.

In 2001, Pfirrmann and colleagues[13] proposed a 5-level grading scale for the evaluation of disc degeneration on T2 SE-WI (**Box 1**).

Before the advent of MR imaging, the reference imaging modality to visualize spinal disc

---

Box 1
Five-level grading scale for evaluating disc degeneration on T2 spin echo–weighted imaging

- *Grade I:* disc is homogeneous with bright hyperintense white signal intensity and normal disc height

- *Grade II:* disc is inhomogeneous, but keeping the hyperintense white signal. Nucleus and *annulus* are clearly differentiated and a horizontal gray band could be present at the central aspect of the disc; eight is normal

- *Grade III:* disc is inhomogeneous with an intermittent gray signal intensity. Distinction between *nucleus* and *annulus* is unclear; disc height is normal or slightly decreased

- *Grade IV:* disc is inhomogeneous with a hypointense dark gray signal intensity. There is no more distinction between the *nucleus* and *annulus*; disc height is slightly or moderately decreased

- *Grade V:* disc is inhomogeneous with a hypointense black signal intensity. There is no more distinction between the *nucleus* and *annulus*; the disc space is collapsed

degeneration was the discography, which consists of the puncture of the intervertebral disc with a needle under fluoroscopic guidance and subsequent injection of contrast material.[14] In the mid 1980s, MR imaging has been shown to be a valuable noninvasive imaging technique to depict disc degeneration, especially for early signs of degeneration like intradiscal fissures.[15] Yu and colleagues[16] have described 3 patterns of intradiscal fissures related to spinal disc degeneration on T2-WI (**Fig. 1**).

Annular fissure is a subtype of disc fissure located within the annulus fibrosus. It appears on T2-WI as a focal high intensity zone within the annulus (most commonly in its peripheral aspect).[17] According to a recent recommendation for lumbar disc degeneration nomenclature,[18] the term "fissure" should be used instead of "tear" because tear has a connotation of injury.

When disc degeneration is evolved, it may lead to disc bulging or even herniation when the disc loses its cohesion and its mechanical properties. Sometimes, major disc degeneration may appear as intradiscal gas (most frequently nitrogen) or may lead to disc calcification (appearing in both conditions as hypointense signals on T1-WI and T2-WI).

DISC HERNIATION

Disc protrusion or extrusion consists of focal bulging of disc material (nucleus, annulus, and/or material from the endplate). Disc protrusion or extrusion has the same signal as the intervertebral disc. Sometimes, the protrusion or herniation may appear with a hyperintense signal on T2-WI. Peripheral enhancement may be seen after contrast media injection, especially in the lumbar region, and may be related to inflammatory processes, neovascularization, or both (**Fig. 2**).[19] This inflammation-related enhancement should be distinguished from the epidural venous plexus. This inflammatory process may help to resorb spontaneously the disc herniation.

The terminology for intervertebral disc bulging is very muddled.[20] The most widely used nomenclature is as follows (**Fig. 3**)[18,21]:

- *Disc bulging*: circumferential (symmetric or asymmetric) disc enlargement.
- *Disc herniation*: disc protrusion or extrusion leading to a focal bulging, usually 3 mm or greater, beyond the vertebral margin.
- *Disc protrusion*: eccentric herniation with a broad-based connection with disc (the greatest distance, in any plane, between the edges of

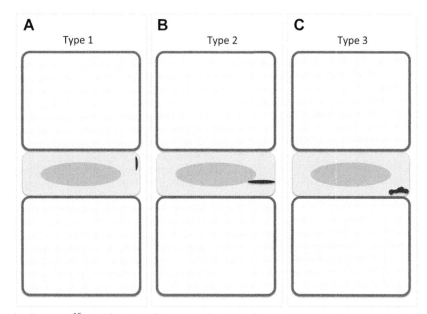

Fig. 1. Yu and colleagues'[16] classification of intervertebral disc fissures. (*A*) Type 1: concentric fissure. (*B*) Type 2: radial fissure. (*C*) Type 3: transverse fissure. Type 1 concentric fissures are related to the rupture of the short transverse fibers that connect the lamellae composing the annulus. They appear as crescentic or oval hyperintensities filled with fluid or mucoid material within the disc. Type 2 radial fissures are related to disruption of the longitudinal fibers through all layers of the annulus (from the peripheral aspect of the annulus to the nucleus). Type 3 transverse fissures are owing to rupture of Sharpey's fibers near their attachments with the ring apophysis. They appear as irregular, fluid-filled cavities at the peripheral aspect of the annulus.

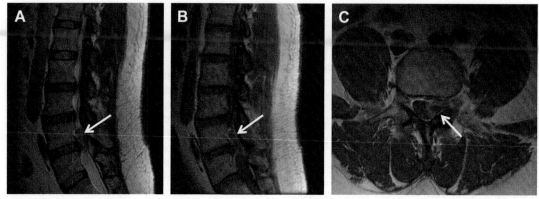

Fig. 2. Lumbar MR imaging. Sagittal T2-weighted imaging (WI); (*A*) and contrast-enhanced T1-WI (*B*). Axial contrast-enhanced T1-WI on L4-L5 level (*C*). Example of peripheral enhancement surrounding a cranially migrated disc herniation (*arrows*).

the disc material beyond the disc space is less than the distance between the edges of the base in the same plane).

- *Disc extrusion*: eccentric disc bulging with a narrowed connection to the disc.
- *Free fragment*: epidural fragment of disc inside the vertebral canal with no connection to the intervertebral disc. This pattern may also be called "*sequestration*." The free fragment is located more frequently at the anterior aspect of the spinal canal, but may also be observed at the lateral or even posterior aspect of the canal (**Fig. 4**). A free fragment in the intradural compartment may be observed rarely, when the

disc fragment has ruptured through the thecal sac.

- *Migration*: disc herniation with upward or downward migration compared with the disc's plane (**Fig. 5**).
- *Contained disc herniation*: the displaced part of the disc is covered by the outer fibers of the annulus fibrosus and/or by the PLL. This pattern of herniation is also called "subligamentous herniation."
- *Uncontained disc herniation*: the herniated fragment is neither covered by the peripheral aspect of the annulus nor by the PLL.
- *Transligamentous disc herniation*: disc extrusion through the PLL.

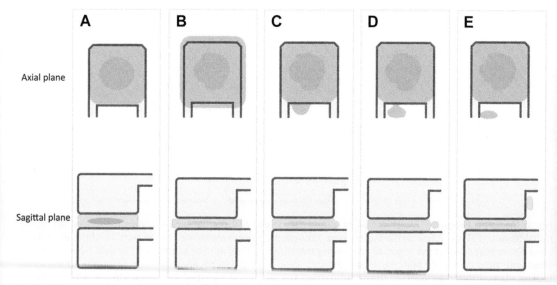

Fig. 3. Different pattern of disc bulging/herniation. Upper row, upper view; lower row, lateral view. (*A*) Normal pattern. (*B*) Symmetric disc bulging. (*C*) Disc protrusion. (*D*) Disc extrusion. (*E*) Free fragment.

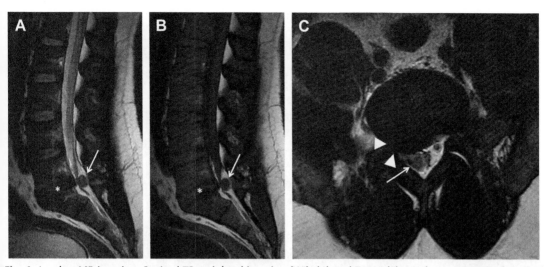

Fig. 4. Lumbar MR imaging. Sagittal T2-weighted imaging (WI); (*A*) and T1-WI (*B*). Moderate L4-L5, and marked L5-S1 disc degeneration (*asterisks*) are seen. (*C*) Axial T2-WI at L5-S1 level. Posterior right L5-S1 disc bulging (*C*, *arrow* heads) associated with a posterior free fragment (sequestration; *white arrows*).

- *Transmembranous disc herniation*: disc extrusion through the peridural membrane.

Most of the disc herniations are located at the lower lumbar spine (L4-L5 and L5-S1). Indeed, the 2 above-mentioned levels account for approximately 90% of disc herniations.[22] On the cervical spine, disc degenerations are usually located at its inferior aspect (ie, C5-C6 and C6-C7 levels). It is noteworthy that thoracic spine disc herniations are rare (approximately 1%[23]) owing to specific anatomic factors like the low weight of the thoracic intervertebral disc. Disc fragment calcifications are more frequent in the thoracic region than in the cervical or lumbar spine (**Fig. 6**).

Disc bulging or herniation may be responsible for nerve root compression either in the spinal canal (at its lateral aspect: the lateral recess; **Fig. 7**A), in the intervertebral foramen (**Fig. 7**B), or after the exit of the nerve root from the intervertebral foramen (ie, the area lateral to the facet joint).[24] The risk of nerve root compression by disc herniation may be increased by a hypertrophy of the adjacent facet joint, particularly the superior articular process. Nerve root impingement may appear as a simple contact between the disc and the nerve root with loss of the periradicular cerebrospinal fluid (CSF) signal and/or disappearance of the anterior epidural fat's hyperintense signal. In some cases, the nerve root may be pushed back by the herniated disc or even not visible anymore. Increasing size of the nerve root as well as nerve root enhancement (related to

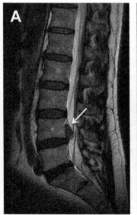
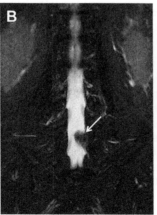
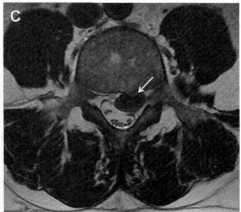

Fig. 5. Lumbar MR imaging. Sagittal T2 (*A*), coronal short tau inversion recovery-weighted imaging (WI); (*B*) and axial T2-WI (*C*) showing an L4-L5 upward migrated disc herniation (*arrows*).

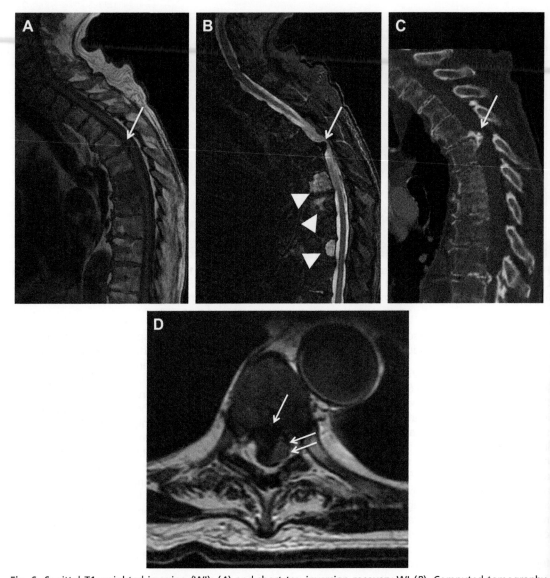

Fig. 6. Sagittal T1-weighted imaging (WI); (*A*) and short tau inversion recovery-WI (*B*). Computed tomography scan of the spine; sagittal reconstruction (*D*). Axial T2-WI at the T4-T5 level. Calcified disc herniation at the T4 to T5 level (*A–D, arrows*), responsible for spinal cord compression (*D, double arrow*). Note multiple spine metastases (*B, arrow heads*).

breakdown of the blood–nerve barrier and to changes in capillary permeability of the nerve root[25]) are radiological signs of nerve root suffering in case of compressive disc herniation.[26] Rarely, an osteophyte may be responsible for nerve root compression. Disc herniation or bulging may also be responsible for spinal cord irritation or compression or for cauda equina syndrome in case of major disc herniation below the conus medullaris (**Fig. 8**).

The pathomechanisms involved in radioulopathy may be a direct compression of the nerve root by the herniated disc and/or related to inflammatory reaction around the herniated disc, leading to an irritation of the nerve root.[27]

Disc degeneration is associated in more than one-half of the cases with changes of the vertebral endplates adjacent to the diseased disc.[28]

The intervertebral disc participates for the congruency of a true articulation between the endplates of 2 adjacent vertebral bodies. As for other joints of the body with arthrosis, degeneration of the cartilaginous endplates (fissures) leading to edematous reaction of the subchondral bone marrow may be observed in disc degenerative disease. In 1988, Modic and colleagues[29]

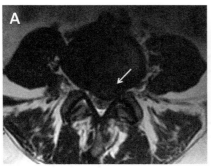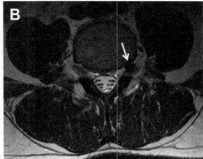

Fig. 7. Different types of nerve root compression related to disc herniation displayed by axial T2-weighted imaging. (A) Nerve root compression inside the vertebral canal (arrow). (B) Nerve root compression by disc material inside the intervertebral foramen (free fragment; arrow).

detailed the subchondral bone marrow changes on MR imaging acquisitions in discarthrosis, and have subdivided the signal changes into 3 patterns (**Figs. 9** and **10**).

Modic Type 1

Modic type 1 changes includes an inflammatory reaction with bone marrow edema and vascular congestion. It appears as a hypointense signal on T1-WI and hyperintense signal on T2-WI and STIR-WI. Enhancement is observed commonly after gadolinium injection. Sometimes, Modic's type 1 inflammatory changes may be so pronounced that they may mimic a spondylodiscitis.[30] However, when increased disc signal intensity on T2-WI and/or paravertebral or epidural abscess are seen, the more likely diagnosis is an infectious spondylitis rather than Modic type 1 degeneration.[31]

Modic Type 2

Modic type 2 inflammation entails subchondral fatty conversion of the bone marrow. These changes appear as a hyperintense signal on both T1-WI and T2-WI, and hypointense on STIR-WI. Type 2 changes may be observed as frequently as in 20% of the cases in patients greater than 50 years of age, and are usually located in the anterior one-third of the vertebral endplate.[32]

Modic Type 3

Modic type 3 changes include sclerotic changes of the subchondral bone marrow. They appear as hypointense signal on T1-WI, T2-WI, and STIR-WI.

Evolution from Modic's type 1 to type 3 usually takes a few years of time. Some congenital vertebral anomalies, like lumbosacral transitional vertebrae, may favor disc degeneration.[33]

DEGENERATIVE SPINAL STENOSIS

Spinal stenoses correspond with a decrease in the spinal canal's surface; they are divided into congenital and acquired stenoses. Among acquired spinal stenoses, degenerative condition is the most frequent etiology.[34] The reduction of the spinal canal surface in degenerative stenoses is caused by thickening, herniation, or migration

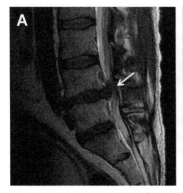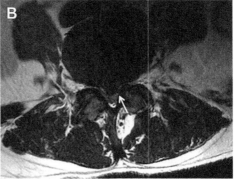

Fig. 8. Lumbar spine MR imaging. Sagittal T2-weighted image (WI); (A) and axial T2-WI (B). Median L4-L5 disc herniation responsible for a compression of the cauda equina in the lumbar canal (A and B, arrows).

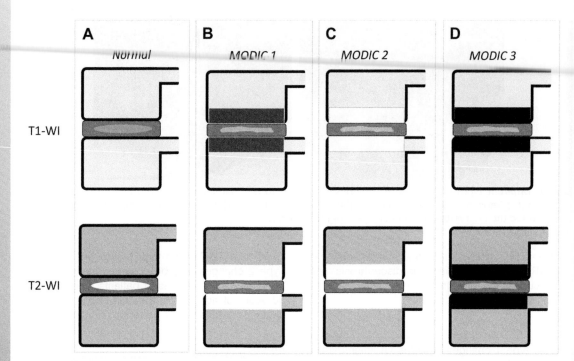

Fig. 9. Different patterns of medullar bone changes in discarthrosis according to Modic and colleagues' classification. Upper row, T1-weighted images (WI); lower row, T2-WI. (*A*) Normal pattern. (*B*) Modic type 1 (inflammatory changes). (*C*) Modic type 2 (fatty changes). (*D*) Modic type 3 (sclerotic changes). (*Data from* Modic MT, Steinberg PM, Ross JS, et al. Degenerative disk disease: assessment of changes in vertebral body marrow with MR imaging. Radiology 1988;166:193–9.)

of materials surrounding the spinal canal, which may be worsened by a spondylolisthesis. Severe spinal stenosis may be responsible for compression of the neural components inside the canal, leading to neurologic symptoms. In contrast with congenital stenosis, which is owing to short pedicles, acquired spinal stenosis is related to degenerative changes associating facet joints hypertrophy, intracanal disc bulging or herniation, and/or thickening of the ligamentum flavum. Both congenital and acquired mechanisms can be associated.[34] Spinal stenoses are observed more frequently at the cervical and lumbar levels. However, spinal stenoses at both levels can be associated at the same time.[35] MR imaging is the best modality to demonstrate accurately the surface reduction of the spinal canal.[36,37] However, CT scan, by displaying more precisely the bone landmarks of the spinal canal, may be more appropriate to explore congenital canal stenosis.

Cervical Stenosis

Clinically, cervical canal stenosis will carry neurologic symptoms that may involve both the inferior and the upper limbs (pyramidal syndrome, motor, and/or sensory deficits).[38] Symptoms related to

cervical stenosis thus may include: numbness of the hands or clumsiness, arm or hand weakness, arm or hand hypoesthesia, or leg stiffness. Even if neck pain is usually present, it is frequently not the prevalent symptom. The pathophysiology of cervical spine stenosis is not understood completely. It is thought to be multifactorial, associating static factors responsible for spine canal constriction and repetitive injuries to the spinal cord.[39] Cervical spinal stenosis is usually related to multilevel disc bulging or herniations at the mid and lower cervical region that will reduce the anterior perimedullary space (which appears as a thinning down or disappearance of the CSF hyperintense signal on T2-WI).[40] Most of the time, these bulging/herniations are associated with a thickening of the ligamenta flava leading to a reduction of the posterior perimedullary space and hypertrophy of the uncus processes owing to arthrosis responsible for lateral and/or anterior spine canal stenosis. Cervical canal stenosis may increase in hyperextension owing to a bulging of the ligamentum flavum secondary to tension release (**Fig. 11**). Thus, open MR imaging allowing for exploration of the cervical spine in flexion and extension may help to depict more accurately a cervical spinal stenosis.[41]

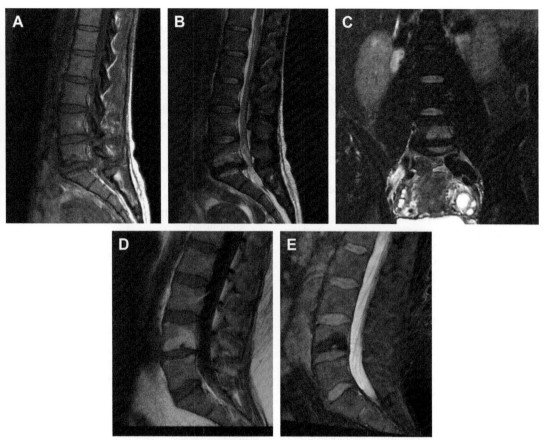

Fig. 10. (*A–C*) MR imaging pattern of Modic 1 changes. Lumbar spine MR imaging; sagittal T1-weighted image (WI); (*A*) and T2-WI (*B*). Coronal short tau inversion recovery (STIR)-WI (*C*). Hypointense signal of endplates surrounding the L5-S1 degenerative disc on T1-WI (*A*); hyperintense signal of the bone marrow on both T2 and STIR-WI (*B* and *C*). (*D, E*) MR imaging pattern of Modic 2 changes. Hyperintense signal of the L4 inferior endplate is seen on T1-WI (*A*), corresponding with a hypointense signal area on T2 fat saturated WI (*B*), suggestive of fatty changes.

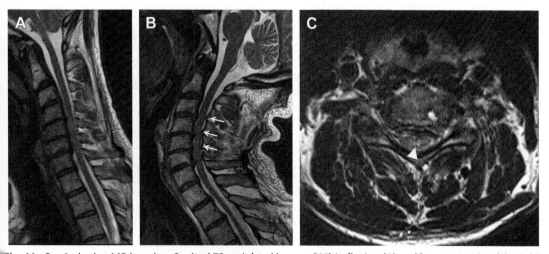

Fig. 11. Cervical spine MR imaging. Sagittal T2-weighted images (WI) in flexion (*A*) and hyperextension (*B*). Multi-level cervical spine disc protrusions associated with hypertrophy of the ligamenta flava are seen, responsible for cervical spine stenosis. Note the increasing of the stenosis in hyperextension owing to the bulging of the *ligamenta flava* (*B, arrows*). (*C*). Axial T2-WI showing a hyperintense signal within the spinal cord, corresponding to a myelopathy (*arrowhead*).

Imaging absolute size criteria for cervical spine stenosis are very difficult to define owing to great interindividual variability.[36,42] Thus, the diagnosis of cervical spine stenosis should be retained only taking into account patient's history, clinical symptoms, and imaging findings. Grading scales may, however, help in evaluating the severity of the cervical spine stenosis.[43]

Myelopathy owing to compression by the protruding material inside the cervical canal appears as a hyperintense signal on T2-WI within the cervical spinal cord at the level where the cord impingement is maximal (see **Fig. 11**). This hyperintense signal may be related to inflammation, edema, ischemia, gliosis, or myelomalacia.[39] It usually corresponds with an irreversible medullary lesion. However, the lack of this hyperintensity within the spinal cord does not rule out a myelopathy. Finally, diffusion-weighted imaging and tensor diffusion imaging may be interesting tools to depict early spinal cord lesions,[44] but are not at this time used in regular clinical practice.

Lumbar Stenosis

Clinically, lumbar stenosis should be suspected in patients with neurogenic intermittent claudication. Neurogenic intermittent claudication is provoked by prolonged standing or lumbar extension and resolves with sitting, lying, or trunk flexion/stooped position. These clinical symptoms are believed to be related to venous congestion and hypertension of the nerve roots owing to the spinal canal constriction. Associated with neurogenic intermittent claudication, back pain and sciatica may be observed in as many as 95% of the cases.[45] Lumbar stenosis affects predominantly patients greater than 70 years of age and more frequently women.[46]

Numerous attempts have been made to provide standard measurement to define lumbar stenosis.[47] For instance, an anteroposterior diameter on CT acquisition of less than 10 mm has been proposed as criterion for lumbar stenosis.[48] However, there are a lot of false-positive diagnoses using only measurement criteria.[49]

Spine MR imaging is the standard imaging technique for the demonstration of lumbar stenosis. Its sensitivity is as high as 96%, but its specificity is only about 70% to 75%.[50] MR imaging patterns in lumbar stenosis associate a reduction of the thecal sac's size (by disc bulging or herniations anteriorly, thickening of the ligamenta flava posteriorly, and hypertrophy of the facet joints laterally). An associated spondylolisthesis secondary to severe facet joint arthrosis may be observed and worsens the lumbar stenosis. The nerve roots of the cauda equina may present an accordion shape

that seen is more easily on sagittal T2-WI (**Fig. 12**). Finally, a periradicular enhancement may also be seen, which is thought to be related to congestion. A grading scale has been proposed by Schizas and colleagues[51] (**Fig. 13**) to evaluate the severity of the lumbar stenosis as follows:

A. CSF is clearly visible inside the thecal sac, but its distribution is inhomogeneous.
B. Some CSF is still present giving a grainy appearance to the thecal sac. The rootlets occupy the whole of the dural sac, but they can still be individualized.
C. The dural sac demonstrating a homogeneous gray signal with no CSF. No rootlets can be recognized.
D. In addition to no rootlets being recognizable, there is no epidural fat posteriorly.

FACET JOINT ARTHROSIS

Lumbar facet joint or zygapophyseal osteoarthritis is common and represents a major source of neck

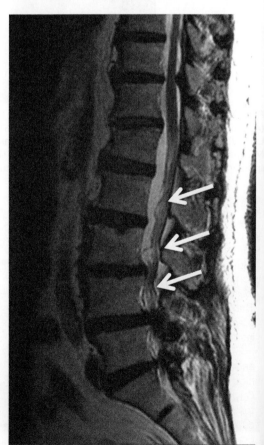

Fig. 12. Lumbar spine MR imaging. Sagittal T2-weighted image showing the irregular shape of the nerve roots inside the lumbar canal (*arrows*) in a case of lumbar severe stenosis.

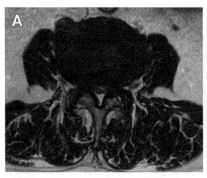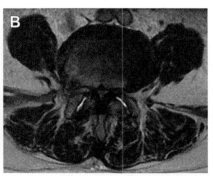

Fig. 13. Lumbar spine MR imaging in 2 different patients with lumbar stenosis. Axial T2-weighted image (*A*) Schizas type C[51] spinal stenosis with undistinguishable rootlets and no visible cerebrospinal fluid. (*B*) Very tight Schizas type D[51] spinal stenosis in another patient. No cerebrospinal fluid and no posterior epidural fat are visible. In both cases, note the zygapophyseal osteoarthritis and hypertrophic ligamentum flavum contributing to the thecal sac stenosis in conjunction with the disc bulging.

and low back pain. It may account for 15% to 40% of low back pain.[52] Facet joints are an important source of symptoms because of high-level mobility and load forces, especially in the lumbar area.[53] They play an important role in load transmission stabilizing the spine in flexion and extension and restricting axial rotation. Degenerative changes in the facet joint comprise cartilage degradation that leads to the formation of focal and then diffuse erosions with joint space narrowing and sclerosis of the subchondral bone. Facet joint osteoarthritis results from a complex multifactorial process closely intertwined with intervertebral discs degeneration.[54] The capsule of the facet joint, subchondral bone and synovium are richly innervated and can be a potential source of low back pain.[53]

Facet joints have a biomechanical role of facilitating articulation of the vertebra. They are diarthrodial synovial joints with opposing articular cartilage. Together with the disc, the bilateral facet joints transfer loads, and guide and constrain motions in the spine.[55] The facet joints transmit shear forces and carry about 16% of the vertical load.[56] The orientation of the lumbar facet joints allows greater flexion motion and prevents rotatory instability.

Biomechanical studies have shown that lumbar and cervical facet joint capsules can undergo high strains during spine loading.[57] According to Cavanaugh and colleagues,[57] inflammation leads to decreased thresholds of nerve endings in facet capsules and increased baseline discharge rates. For instance, rear-end motor vehicle impacts can cause excessive deformation of the capsules of lower cervical facet joints. This deformation may activate nociceptors and lead to prolonged neural discharges, causing persistent neck pain.

Both cervical and lumbar facet syndromes have been described in the medical literature. At the neck level, it predominates at the C3 to C6 level. It is rare at the thoracic level because of restricted mobility.

At the lumbar level, it is often associated with disc degeneration and canal narrowing.[58] Osteophytes develop preferentially at the anteromedial aspect of the joint. Radicular pains may be triggered by irritation of the ascending nerve root. Spine physicians diagnose zygapophyseal joint pain on analgesic response to anesthetic injections into the zygapophyseal joints.[59]

Additionally, facet joint osteoarthritis may be responsible for instability and spondylolisthesis. Degenerative spondylolisthesis is defined as an anterior vertebral slipping of a vertebra on the immediate lower vertebra in the sagittal plane with an intact neural arch, as opposed to isthmic spondylolisthesis.[60] It can be observed at lumbar or cervical level (**Fig. 14**). Risk factors for lumbar facet joint osteoarthritis include advanced age, more sagittal orientation of the facet joint, and a background of intervertebral disc degeneration.

Facet joint osteoarthritis imaging semiology is similar to other locations, that is, joint space narrowing, osteophytes, subchondral erosions, bone sclerosis, and sometimes effusion. It is, however, often characterized by the predominance of osteophytes with a hypertrophy of the articular masses (**Fig. 15**). Another characteristic is the hypertrophy and calcifications of the ligamenta flava. A hypertrophic facet joint with prominent osteophytes can cause intervertebral foramen narrowing that may lead to radicular pain (**Fig. 16**). They may also reduce the interdisc apophyseal passes and cause conflict with the emergences of the nerve roots before they enter the foramina.

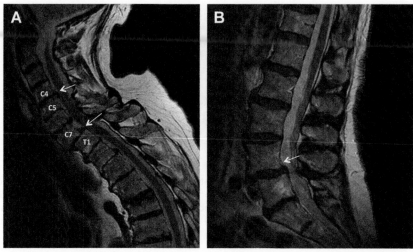

Fig. 14. (*A*) Sagittal T2-weighted image (WI) of the cervical spine showing multiple degenerative anterolisthesis: slip of C4 on C5 and C7 on T1 (*arrows*). (*B*) Sagittal T2-WI view of a lumbar spine MR (other patient) showing intervertebral disc degeneration, interspinous osteoarthritis and zygapophyseal arthrosis (not presented) causing sagittal instability with anterior slip of L4 on L5 (*arrow*).

Synovial Cysts

Zygapophyseal cysts are secondary to arthrosis degeneration of articular cavities and development of a neocavity. Both anterior and posterior lumbar facet joint synovial cysts are rare. Posterior cysts are more common than anterior cysts (**Fig. 17**). Both types of cysts are related to facet joint osteoarthritis, but not to disc disease.[61] They are much more rare at the neck level. Anterior cysts develop within the spinal canal and can cause conflict with the nerve roots. Lumbar facet joint cysts occurrence is associated with higher rates of arthritis and coronally orientated facet joint.[62]

Facet Joint Effusion

Facet joint fluid effusion is not specific for osteoarthritis and can be observed in young and healthy patients without facet joint degeneration. However, facet joint effusion is a frequent finding in association with osteoarthritis and could be a sign of micromotions (**Fig. 18**). According to some authors, if thickness is greater than 1.5 mm, facet fluid effusion could be predictive of degenerative spondylolisthesis at the L4-L5 level, even in the absence of measurable anterolisthesis on supine MR imaging. In this condition, they recommend standing lateral flexion–extension plain radiographs.[63]

MR Imaging of Facet Joint Osteoarthritis

Because the most prominent changes occur in bone, CT scan can be considered as the best imaging technique for evaluation of the facet joint.[53] Indeed, CT scan provides a better evaluation of bony changes and is more accurate in quantifying bone sclerosis and measure cartilage thinning,[64] and MR may underestimate the severity of facet joint osteoarthritis. However, several studies have

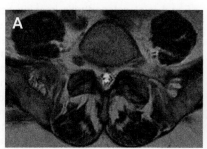
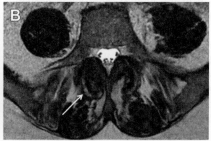

Fig. 15. (*A*) Axial T2 weighted image (WI) of lumbar spine showing bilateral facet joints osteoarthritis at the L5-S1 level, predominating on the right side with joint space narrowing, bone sclerosis, and hypertrophic osteophytes. (*B*) Evolved bilateral L5-L1 facet joint osteoarthritis with exuberant "wrap around bumper" osteophyte formations (*arrow*), providing a stabilizing effect.

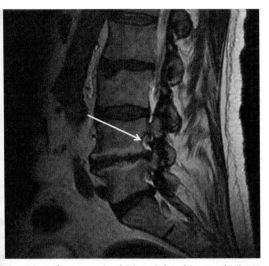

Fig. 16. Left parasagittal T2-weighted image (WI) MR acquisition of the lumbar spine. Evolved L4-L5 intervertebral disc degeneration associated with facet joint osteoarthritis. Prominent osteophytes inside the foramina can cause formaminal stenosis (*arrow*). At an advanced stage, foraminal stenosis may cause nerve root irritation.

shown a good to excellent agreement between CT and MR imaging to assess facet joint degeneration[64,65] and MR imaging has proven to be an excellent method to evaluate the whole spine on the same examination. Moreover, MR imaging is superior to detect congestive edema, facet effusion, and cysts, especially on STIR or T2 fat saturation sequences (**Fig. 19**). MR imaging can also bring information not only of morphologic changes, but also pathologic changes of osteoligamentous and neural components.[66] Fujiwara and colleagues[64] have proposed a 4-grade classification from 1 to 4: grade 1, normal; grade 2, joint space narrowing or mild osteophyte; grade 3, sclerosis or moderate osteophyte; and grade 4, marked osteophyte. Additionally, these authors described the "wraparound bumper" osteophyte formations along the capsular attachments of the facet joint, providing an additional stabilizing effect in segmental degenerative disease (see **Fig. 15B**).

Risk Factors

A sagittal orientation of facet joints is associated to osteoarthritis of the lumbar facet joint.[67] The

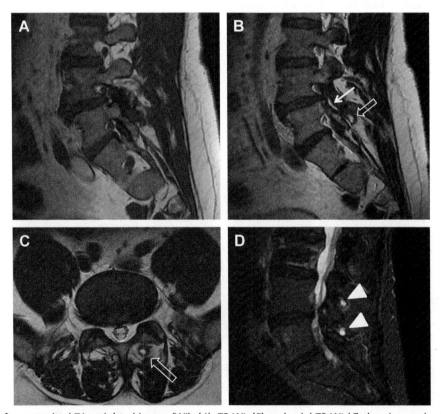

Fig. 17. Left parasagittal T1-weighted image (WI); (*A*), T2-WI, (*B*) and axial T2-WI (*C*) showing evolved left L4-L5 facet joint osteoarthritis with facet effusion (*arrow*) and a small posterior synovial cyst (*hollow arrows*). (*D*) Left parasagittal short tau inversion recovery sequence in another patient showing facet joint osteoarthritis and 2 posterior zygapophysial cysts at the L3-L4 and L4-L5 levels (*arrowheads*).

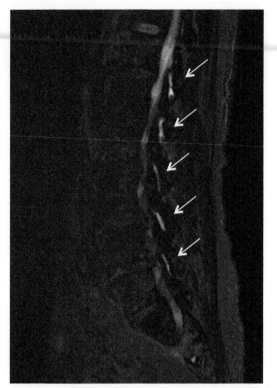

Fig. 18. Lumbar spine MR in short tau inversion recovery sequence, right parasagittal view, showing facet joint osteoarthritis and facet joint effusion at all lumbar levels (*arrows*). Effusion appears hyperintense, whereas the fat signal is suppressed.

coronal and flat orientation in the lower lumbar spine to resist against flexion and shearing forces.[56] The facet angle is measured relative to the coronal plane. A more coronally oriented facet joint— 60° of greater at the upper lumbar spine—may be an individual risk factor for the development of facet joint arthritis.[56] In the lower spine, a larger mean facet angle measured is also associated with degenerative spondylolisthesis, with a threshold of 45°.[36] Wang and Yang[68] have found that a coronal orientation of L4 and L5 was associated with advanced age, suggesting this could explain why elderly people are more prone to degenerative spondylolisthesis. Long-evolved facet joint osteoarthritis may result in joint fusion and ankylosis, which generally stops the pain (**Fig. 20**).

Treatment

Anesthetics and corticosteroid infiltrations are interesting for both diagnostic and therapeutic purposes. Other more invasive techniques like percutaneous thermocoagulation can be performed.[58] Facet joint osteoarthritis can also be treated by lumbar spinal fusion. However, although spinal fusion generally helps in eliminating certain types of pain, it may also decrease function by limiting mobility.[69] Furthermore, fusion may increase stresses on adjacent vertebral mobile segments, accelerating their degeneration. Total joint replacement with facet arthroplasty of the lumbar spine represents a new insight in spine surgery.

INTERSPINOUS PROCESSES ARTHROSIS

Interspinous processes arthrosis, also known as Baastrup disease or "kissing spine" is less

orientation of the facet joints varies according to their levels. Whereas they have a more sagittal and curved orientation in the upper lumbar spine to resist against axial rotation, they have a more

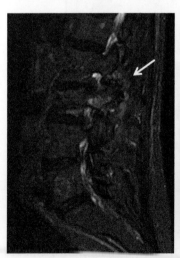
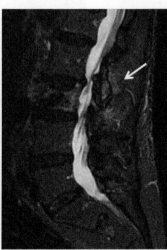
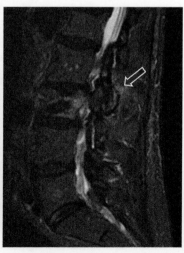

Fig. 19. Short tau inversion recovery sequence, left parasagittal views showing hypertrophic L2-L3 facet joint osteoarthritis. Hyperintensity of bone and periarticular tissues reflects congestive edema (*arrows*). Note the presence of a small posterior facet joint synovial cyst (*hollow arrow*).

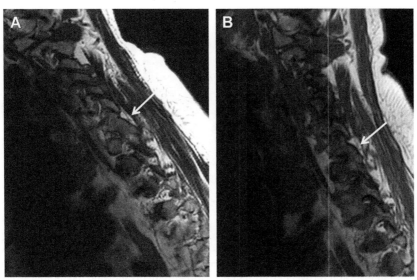

Fig. 20. Left parasagittal MR of the cervicothoracic spine in T2-weighted image (WI); (*A*) and T1-WI (*B*). Evolved facet joint osteoarthritis eventually led to bone fusion and ankylosis of the left C7-T1 facet joint (*arrows*) with loss of joint mobility.

common than facet joint osteoarthritis. It was described first by Baastrup C in 1933 in the lumbar spine.[70] It results from abnormal contact between 2 spinous processes with development of sclerosis, enlargement, and flattening of the spinous processes and causes back pain. Very few cases of Baastrup disease have been described at cervical level.[71] No report exists at thoracic level.

Typical clinical symptoms are low back pain that increases with extension and is relieved in flexion of the lumbar back in a characteristic position.[72] Clinical examination finds a pain when pressing the interspinous space.

Frequency increases with advancing age with a peak in patients greater than 80 years of age. Associated degenerative changes (disc degeneration, spondylolisthesis, and facet joint osteoarthritis) are almost constantly associated.[73] It is poorly studied and few data exist concerning the epidemiology of Baastrup disease.[74] In a cohort of 539 patients undergoing lumbar MR imaging, Maes and associates[75] have reported a prevalence of Baastrup disease of 8.2%, associated with advanced age, central canal stenosis, disc bulging, and anterolisthesis. Baastrup disease can be responsible for some cases of radicular pain.

Mechanical constraints enter into account in the genesis of this disease, especially in a professional context. For instance, a greater prevalence of Baastrup disease has been reported in professional heavy motor vehicle operators, with a predominant involvement of the L3-L4 and L4-L5 levels.[76]

Pathophysiology

Interspinous osteoarthrosis, hyperlordosis, and ligament destruction by compression are the main inducing factors. The soft interspinous tissue lesions and the presence of neosynovium-lined joints or interspinous bursitis are known by cadaver dissections. On MR imaging, interspinous bursitis is visible as a concave up liquid signal between consecutive spinous processes hypointense in T1-WI and hyperintense in T2-WI (**Fig. 21**).

Risk factors for Baastrup disease are an excessive lumbar lordosis, large spinous processes, or a small interspinous space owing to disc space narrowing or vertebral fracture. When interspinous tissues are destroyed, the adjacent spinous processes come in contact over a small surface causing osteoarthritis changes. Radiologic signs are marginal sclerosis, a faceted aspect of the processes, osteophytes, and bony erosions. On MR imaging, subchondral edema and bursitis can be observed (see **Fig. 21**; **Fig. 22**). At a late stage, ankylosis can be seen.

Interspinous bursitis may represent an early stage of the disease. It consists of interspinous neojoints with synovial membrane, cartilage, and a fibrous capsule. Moreover, an

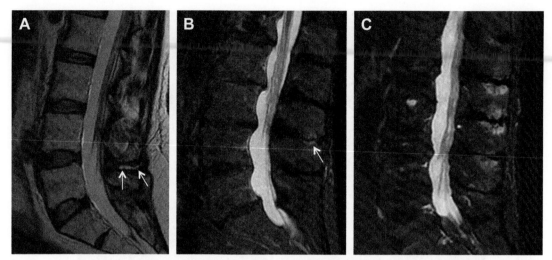

Fig. 21. MR image of the lumbar spine in T2-weighted image sagittal sequence (*A*) showing interspinous bursitis (*arrows*). (*B*) Short tau inversion recovery (STIR) sequence (other patient) showing moderate L3-L4 Baastrup disease–associated interspinous contact, bony erosions, and a slight subchondral bone edema (*arrow*). Note the multilevel disc degeneration and disc space narrowing causing interspinous contact. (*C*) STIR sagittal sequence (other patient) showing multilevel interspinous osteoarthritis with marked bony erosions and subchondral edema. Baastrup disease is most likely secondary to the multiple vertebral bodies fractures causing loss of height and narrowing of interspinous spaces.

interspinous bursitis is sometimes filled during facet joint arthrography. Interspinous bursitis creates a communication between one facet joint and the contralateral facet joint. Bursography followed by infiltration is technically easy.

Baastrup osteoarthritis can be treated conservatively or surgically. If clinical findings are compatible and if there is no other cause for low back pain, late-acting steroid injection guided by opacification of the bursal space can be performed and may produce pain relief. There have been case reports of iatrogenic Baastrup disease resulting from anterior lumbar surgery. Some authors suggest spinous process excision to prevent this complication.[72]

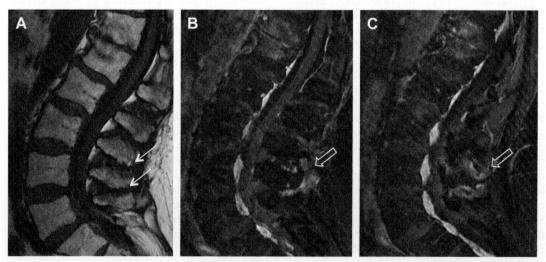

Fig. 22. MR image of the lumbar spine in sagittal T1-weighted imaging (WI); (*A*) and T1-WI with fat saturation after gadolinium injection (*B* and *C*) showing marked L3-L4 and L4-L5 Baastrup osteoarthritis. Interspinous contact, bony erosions, and subchondral condensation are well visible (*arrows*). After contrast, there is a peripheral enhancement of interspinous bursitis and of inflammatory peripheral tissues (*hollow arrows*). Note the increased lumbar lordosis most likely responsible for Baastrup disease.

REFERENCES

1. Endean A, Palmer KT, Coggon D. Potential of magnetic resonance imaging findings to refine case definition for mechanical low back pain in epidemiological studies: a systematic review. Spine (Phila Pa 1976) 2011;36:160–9.
2. Malhotra A, Kalra VB, Wu X, et al. Imaging of lumbar spinal surgery complications. Insights Imaging 2015;6:579–90.
3. Jones KM, Unger EC, Granstrom P, et al. Bone marrow imaging using STIR at 0.5 and 1.5 T. Magn Reson Imaging 1992;10:169–76.
4. Bakar B, Sumer MM, Cila A, et al. An extreme lateral lumbar disc herniation mimicking L4 schwannoma. Acta Neurol Belg 2009;109:155–8.
5. Chen CF, Chang MC, Liu CL, et al. Acute noncontiguous multiple-level thoracic disc herniations with myelopathy: a case report. Spine (Phila Pa 1976) 2004;29:E157–60.
6. Roberts S, Evans H, Trivedi J, et al. Histology and pathology of the human intervertebral disc. J Bone Joint Surg Am 2006;88(Suppl 2):10–4.
7. Yu SW, Haughton VM, Lynch KL, et al. Fibrous structure in the intervertebral disk: correlation of MR appearance with anatomic sections. AJNR Am J Neuroradiol 1989;10:1105–10.
8. Raj PP. Intervertebral disc: anatomy-physiology-pathophysiology-treatment. Pain Pract 2008;8:18–44.
9. Bibby SR, Jones DA, Lee RB, et al. The pathophysiology of the intervertebral disc. Joint Bone Spine 2001;68:537–42.
10. Zhao CQ, Wang LM, Jiang LS, et al. The cell biology of intervertebral disc aging and degeneration. Ageing Res Rev 2007;6:247–61.
11. Wang F, Cai F, Shi R, et al. Aging and age related stresses: a senescence mechanism of intervertebral disc degeneration. Osteoarthritis Cartilage 2015; 24(3):398–408.
12. Videman T, Nummi P, Battie MC, et al. Digital assessment of MRI for lumbar disc desiccation. A comparison of digital versus subjective assessments and digital intensity profiles versus discogram and macroanatomic findings. Spine (Phila Pa 1976) 1994;19:192–8.
13. Pfirrmann CW, Metzdorf A, Zanetti M, et al. Magnetic resonance classification of lumbar intervertebral disc degeneration. Spine (Phila Pa 1976) 2001;26: 1873–8.
14. Legre J, Dufour M, Debaene A, et al. Lumbar discography. Value and indications based on 300 examinations. Neurochirurgie 1971;17:559–78 [in French].
15. Modic MT, Pavlicek W, Weinstein MA, et al. Magnetic resonance imaging of intervertebral disk disease. Clinical and pulse sequence considerations. Radiology 1984;152:103–11.
16. Yu SW, Haughton VM, Sether LA, et al. Comparison of MR and diskography in detecting radial tears of the annulus: a postmortem study. AJNR Am J Neuroradiol 1989;10:1077–81.
17. Schellhas KP, Pollei SR, Gundry CR, et al. Lumbar disc high-intensity zone. Correlation of magnetic resonance imaging and discography. Spine (Phila Pa 1976) 1996;21:79–86.
18. Fardon DF, Williams AL, Dohring EJ, et al. Lumbar disc nomenclature: version 2.0: Recommendations of the combined task forces of the North American Spine Society, the American Society of Spine Radiology and the American Society of Neuroradiology. Spine J 2014;14:2525–45.
19. Ross JS, Modic MT, Masaryk TJ, et al. Assessment of extradural degenerative disease with Gd-DTPA-enhanced MR imaging: correlation with surgical and pathologic findings. AJNR Am J Neuroradiol 1989;10:1243–9.
20. Arana E, Royuela A, Kovacs FM, et al. Lumbar spine: agreement in the interpretation of 1.5-T MR images by using the Nordic Modic Consensus Group classification form. Radiology 2010;254: 809–17.
21. Milette PC. The proper terminology for reporting lumbar intervertebral disk disorders. AJNR Am J Neuroradiol 1997;18:1859–66.
22. Jenis LG, An HS. Spine update. Lumbar foraminal stenosis. Spine (Phila Pa 1976) 2000;25:389–94.
23. Carson J, Gumpert J, Jefferson A. Diagnosis and treatment of thoracic intervertebral disc protrusions. J Neurol Neurosurg Psychiatry 1971;34:68–77.
24. Lee CK, Rauschning W, Glenn W. Lateral lumbar spinal canal stenosis: classification, pathologic anatomy and surgical decompression. Spine (Phila Pa 1976) 1988;13:313–20.
25. Crisi G, Carpeggiani P, Trevisan C. Gadolinium-enhanced nerve roots in lumbar disk herniation. AJNR Am J Neuroradiol 1993;14:1379–92.
26. Itoh R, Murata K, Kamata M, et al. Lumbosacral nerve root enhancement with disk herniation on contrast-enhanced MR. AJNR Am J Neuroradiol 1996;17:1619–25.
27. Hasue M. Pain and the nerve root. An interdisciplinary approach. Spine (Phila Pa 1976) 1993;18: 2053–8.
28. de Roos A, Kressel H, Spritzer C, et al. MR imaging of marrow changes adjacent to end plates in degenerative lumbar disk disease. AJR Am J Roentgenol 1987;149:531–4.
29. Modic MT, Steinberg PM, Ross JS, et al. Degenerative disk disease: assessment of changes in vertebral body marrow with MR imaging. Radiology 1988;166:193–9.
30. Hong SH, Choi JY, Lee JW, et al. MR imaging assessment of the spine: infection or an imitation? Radiographics 2009;29:599–612.

31. Tali ET, Gultekin S. Spinal infections. Eur Radiol 2005;15:599–607.

32. Malghem J. IRM de rachis lombaires « asymptoma tiques » étude multicentrique du GETROA. In: Le rachis lombaire dégénératif. Montpellier (France): Sauramps Médical; 1998. p. 119–28.

33. Konin GP, Walz DM. Lumbosacral transitional vertebrae: classification, imaging findings, and clinical relevance. AJNR Am J Neuroradiol 2010;31:1778–86.

34. Arnoldi CC, Brodsky AE, Cauchoix J, et al. Lumbar spinal stenosis and nerve root entrapment syndromes. Definition and classification. Clin Orthop Relat Res 1976;(115):4–5.

35. Choudhury AR, Taylor JC. The cervicolumbar syndrome. Ann R Coll Surg Engl 1980;62:200–2.

36. Boden SD, Davis DO, Dina TS, et al. Abnormal magnetic-resonance scans of the lumbar spine in asymptomatic subjects. A prospective investigation. J Bone Joint Surg Am 1990;72:403–8.

37. Malghem J, Willems X, Vande Berg B, et al. Comparison of lumbar spinal canal measurements on MRI and CT. J Radiol 2009;90:493–7.

38. Lebl DR, Hughes A, Cammisa FP Jr, et al. Cervical spondylotic myelopathy: pathophysiology, clinical presentation, and treatment. HSS J 2011;7:170–8.

39. Meyer F, Borm W, Thome C. Degenerative cervical spinal stenosis: current strategies in diagnosis and treatment. Dtsch Arztebl Int 2008;105:366–72.

40. Kang Y, Lee JW, Koh YH, et al. New MRI grading system for the cervical canal stenosis. AJR Am J Roentgenol 2011;197:W134–40.

41. Gilbert JW, Wheeler GR, Lingreen RA, et al. Open stand-up MRI: a new instrument for positional neuroimaging. J Spinal Disord Tech 2006;19:151–4.

42. Pavlov H, Torg JS, Robie B, et al. Cervical spinal stenosis: determination with vertebral body ratio method. Radiology 1987;164:771–5.

43. Muhle C, Metzner J, Weinert D, et al. Classification system based on kinematic MR imaging in cervical spondylitic myelopathy. AJNR Am J Neuroradiol 1998;19:1763–71.

44. Ries M, Jones RA, Dousset V, et al. Diffusion tensor MRI of the spinal cord. Magn Reson Med 2000;44: 884–92.

45. Amundsen T, Weber H, Nordal HJ, et al. Lumbar spinal stenosis: conservative or surgical management?: A prospective 10-year study. Spine (Phila Pa 1976) 2000;25:1424–35 [discussion: 1435–6].

46. Lee SY, Kim TH, Oh JK, et al. Lumbar stenosis: a recent update by review of literature. Asian Spine J 2015;9:818–28.

47. Andreisek G, Imhof M, Wertli M, et al. A systematic review of semiquantitative and qualitative radiologic criteria for the diagnosis of lumbar spinal stenosis. AJR Am J Roentgenol 2013;201:W735–46.

48. Kalff R, Ewald C, Waschke A, et al. Degenerative lumbar spinal stenosis in older people: current treatment options. Dtsch Arztebl Int 2013;110: 613–23 [quiz: 624].

49. Jensen MC, Brant-Zawadzki MN, Obuchowski N, et al. Magnetic resonance imaging of the lumbar spine in people without back pain. N Engl J Med 1994;331:69–73.

50. Wassenaar M, van Rijn RM, van Tulder MW, et al. Magnetic resonance imaging for diagnosing lumbar spinal pathology in adult patients with low back pain or sciatica: a diagnostic systematic review. Eur Spine J 2012;21:220–7.

51. Schizas C, Theumann N, Burn A, et al. Qualitative grading of severity of lumbar spinal stenosis based on the morphology of the dural sac on magnetic resonance images. Spine (Phila Pa 1976) 2010;35: 1919–24.

52. Beresford ZM, Kendall RW, Willick SE. Lumbar facet syndromes. Curr Sports Med Rep 2010;9:50–6.

53. Kalichman L, Hunter DJ. Lumbar facet joint osteoarthritis: a review. Semin Arthritis Rheum 2007;37:69–80.

54. Varlotta GP, Lefkowitz TR, Schweitzer M, et al. The lumbar facet joint: a review of current knowledge: part 1: anatomy, biomechanics, and grading. Skeletal Radiol 2011;40:13–23.

55. Jaumard NV, Welch WC, Winkelstein BA. Spinal facet joint biomechanics and mechanotransduction in normal, injury and degenerative conditions. J Biomech Eng 2011;133:071010.

56. Jentzsch T, Geiger J, Zimmermann SM, et al. Lumbar facet joint arthritis is associated with more coronal orientation of the facet joints at the upper lumbar spine. Radiol Res Pract 2013; 2013:693971.

57. Cavanaugh JM, Lu Y, Chen C, et al. Pain generation in lumbar and cervical facet joints. J Bone Joint Surg Am 2006;88(Suppl 2):63–7.

58. Cotten A, Vande Berg B. 15ème mises au point en imagerie ostéo-articulaire. Cliniques Universitaires Saint-Luc, Bruxelles; CHRU de Lille; 2015.

59. Dreyer SJ, Dreyfuss PH. Low back pain and the zygapophysial (facet) joints. Arch Phys Med Rehabil 1996;77:290–300.

60. Ferrero E, Simon A-L, Magrino B, et al. Double-level degenerative spondylolisthesis: what is different in the sagittal plane? Eur Spine J 2016. [Epub ahead of print].

61. Doyle AJ, Merrilees M. Synovial cysts of the lumbar facet joints in a symptomatic population: prevalence on magnetic resonance imaging. Spine 2004;29: 874–8.

62. Ening G, Kowoll A, Stricker I, et al. Lumbar juxtafacet joint cysts in association with facet joint orientation, -tropism and -arthritis: a case-control study. Clin Neurol Neurosurg 2015;100:278 81.

63. Chaput C, Padon D, Rush J, et al. The significance of increased fluid signal on magnetic resonance

imaging in lumbar facets in relationship to degenerative spondylolisthesis. Spine 2007;32:1883–7.

64. Fujiwara A, Tamai K, Yamato M, et al. The relationship between facet joint osteoarthritis and disc degeneration of the lumbar spine: an MRI study. Eur Spine J 1999;8:396–401.

65. Weishaupt D, Zanetti M, Boos N, et al. MR imaging and CT in osteoarthritis of the lumbar facet joints. Skeletal Radiol 1999;28:215–9.

66. Taneichi H. Role of MR imaging in the evaluation of low back pain (orthopedic surgeon's view). Semin Musculoskelet Radiol 2001;5:129–31.

67. Fujiwara A, Tamai K, An HS, et al. The relationship between disc degeneration, facet joint osteoarthritis, and stability of the degenerative lumbar spine. J Spinal Disord 2000;13:444–50.

68. Wang J, Yang X. Age-related changes in the orientation of lumbar facet joints. Spine 2009;34:E596–8.

69. Serhan HA, Varnavas G, Dooris AP, et al. Biomechanics of the posterior lumbar articulating elements. Neurosurg Focus 2007;22:E1.

70. Chancelier. Nouveau regard sur l'arthrose de Baastrup. Rachis 1994;6:241–4.

71. Nava P, Seda H. Kissing spine: Baastrup disease; study of 77 cases, including 63 cases of lumbar spine syndrome, 11 cervical and 3 mixed lumbar and cervical forms. Bras Med 1955;69:546–68 [in Portuguese].

72. Yue JJ, Russo GS, Castro CA. Iatrogenic Baastrup's syndrome: a potential complication following anterior interbody lumbar spinal surgery. Int J Spine Surg 2015;9:66.

73. Kwong Y, Rao N, Latief K. MDCT findings in Baastrup disease: disease or normal feature of the aging spine? AJR Am J Roentgenol 2011;196:1156–9.

74. Farinha F, Raínho C, Cunha I, et al. Baastrup's disease: a poorly recognised cause of back pain. Acta Reumatol Port 2015;40:302–3.

75. Maes R, Morrison WB, Parker L, et al. Lumbar interspinous bursitis (Baastrup disease) in a symptomatic population: prevalence on magnetic resonance imaging. Spine 2008;33:E211–5.

76. Hagner W. Baastrup's disease of the lumbar segment of the spine among drivers of heavy motor vehicles. Med Pr 1988;39:65–70 [in Polish].

MR Imaging and Radiographic Imaging of Degenerative Spine Disorders and Spine Alignment

CrossMark

Fabio Galbusera, PhD[a], Alessio Lovi, MD[b],
Tito Bassani, PhD[a], Marco Brayda-Bruno, MD[b],*

KEYWORDS

- Sagittal alignment • Sagittal balance • Pelvic incidence • Spinopelvic parameters
- Compensatory mechanisms

KEY POINTS

- The pelvis is the keystone of spinal alignment.
- Full standing radiographs (posteroanterior and laterolateral views) are necessary for a proper analysis of the spinopelvic alignment.
- The use of MR imaging alone may not be sufficient for correct pre-operative planning, but should be supplemented by the analysis of the global spinal alignment.

DISCUSSION OF PROBLEM

Advances in MR imaging technologies as well as the widening of their availability boosted their use in the diagnosis of spinal disorders and in the pre-operative planning of spine surgeries. As a matter of fact, MR imaging provides excellent contrast between different types of soft tissues as well as a qualitative estimate of the tissue composition, for example, the water and fibrous contents of the intervertebral disc.[1] These qualities undoubtedly allow for improvements in the diagnosis of various degenerative disorders and facilitate the selection of the optimal treatment. Therefore, MR imaging is often considered the imaging modality of choice in the management of many degenerative disorders of the spine, especially if the symptoms seem to be caused by a single or a couple of motion segments.[2]

Besides, the analysis of planar radiographs of adults with spinal disorders has a long and consolidated tradition in the orthopedic community.[3] Even if taking into account the limited capability of standard radiographs in providing clinically valuable information about soft tissues, the excellent imaging quality of bone tissue together with the possibility of assessing the spinal alignment under the action of a physiologic load (typically the standing posture) provides clear advantages with respect to MR imaging, which is inherently limited by a lower resolution and the horizontal posture of the patient. Thus, it is thought that a combined use of the 2 imaging modalities may be advantageous in cases in which both the clinical status of the soft tissues and the spinal alignment must be taken into account in order to conduct an optimal preoperative planning.

In this article, the radiographic spinopelvic parameters that have relevance in the clinical management of adults with spinal disorders are summarized. One case, in which a preoperative

The authors have nothing to disclose.
[a] Laboratory of Biological Structures Mechanics, IRCCS Istituto Ortopedico Galeazzi, via Galeazzi 4, 20161 Milan, Italy; [b] Department of Spine Surgery III, IRCCS Istituto Ortopedico Galeazzi, via Galeazzi 4, 20161 Milan, Italy
* Corresponding author.
E-mail address: marco.brayda@spinecaregroup.it

Magn Reson Imaging Clin N Am 24 (2016) 515–522
http://dx.doi.org/10.1016/j.mric.2016.04.002
1064-9689/16/$ – see front matter © 2016 Elsevier Inc. All rights reserved.

planning based only on MR images would have possibly led to a suboptimal surgical solution, is then presented and discussed in depth.

ANATOMY
Spinopelvic Alignment

In 1992, a radiological article, which had a decisive impact on spine surgery in the 2 following decades, was published.[4] This work introduced for the first time the relationship between the pelvis (through anatomic and functional pelvic parameters) and the sagittal alignment of the spine, and furthermore, the tendency to maintain the body in the most economical position in terms of energy consumption and vertebral strain. The 3 main pelvic parameters that were identified were the pelvic incidence (PI), the pelvic tilt (PT), and the sacral slope (SS) (**Fig. 1**).

PI is the only one of the 3 parameters that has a fixed anatomic value for each individual and is therefore not dependent on the posture; indeed, it is usually referred to as an anatomic parameter. Several studies assessed the distribution of PI in the general population and reported a marked variability.[5–7] PI approximately ranged between 35° and 85°,[8] with a tendency toward an increase during growth.[9] In these studies, patients with lower PI tended to have a flatter profile of the back, especially a lower curvature of the lumbar spine. The wide distribution of PI in the population did not allow for the determination of clear "healthy" and "pathologic" categories, because the spine curvature seemed to be able to adapt efficiently to the various anatomic morphologies of the pelvis.

PT and SS do not have fixed values in a specific patient, but are dependent on the posture.[4] Indeed, a flexion of both hip joints would lead to a decrease of PT and an increase of SS, whereas PI would be not affected. Both parameters tend to change during the life of the subject, especially during childhood.[9]

Other important descriptors of the spinal shape are the regional curvatures, that is, cervical lordosis (CL), thoracic kyphosis (TK), and lumbar lordosis (LL) (**Fig. 2**). The physiologic curvature of the cervical spine is still a matter of debate, because studies reported an absence of lordosis or a small kyphosis in asymptomatic subjects,[10] whereas well-known studies reported a physiologic lordotic range of 15° to 20°.[11] Similarly, TK was shown to have a wide range in asymptomatic subjects, and an average value in the general population of 40°.[8] As mentioned above, the value of LL is strictly dependent on the pelvic morphology, with subjects having high PI showing correspondingly high LL. There is general agreement about the fact that there is a strong interplay between the regional curvatures of the spine as well as with the pelvis morphology, and a correct analysis of each of these parameters cannot disregard the other regional curvatures.[3]

In order to characterize the global sagittal spinal alignment, other radiological parameters have been introduced and are currently widely used (see **Fig. 2**). The sagittal vertical axis (SVA), also named C7 plumb line, describes the distance in the horizontal direction between a vertical line through the vertebral body of C7 and the postero-superior corner of the sacral plate.[12] SVA is commonly used to describe with a single measurement the global sagittal alignment of the thoracolumbar spine. Values less than 5 cm have been reported as physiologic, whereas higher SVAs characterize sagittal malalignment.[12] It should however be noted that SVA is not a strictly anatomic parameter, but depends on posture.

The difference between PI and LL (PI − LL) is also often used as a single descriptor of the spinal alignment.[13,14] As LL should adapt to the pelvic morphology (described with PI), an excessive mismatch between the 2 values would represent a condition in which the patient is not able to find a spinopelvic organization fitting well her or his pelvic anatomy. It was suggested that a value of PI − LL lower than 10° would indicate a problematic alignment,[13] although the same investigators indicated that this rule should not be interpreted

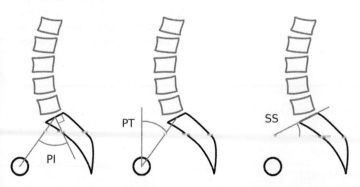

Fig. 1. Definition of the pelvic parameters.

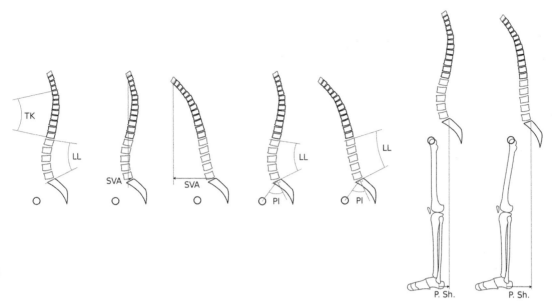

Fig. 2. Radiological parameters used for the evaluation of the sagittal alignment of the spine. From left to right: TK; LL; 2 examples of SVA in a well-aligned and an imbalanced spine; 2 examples: PI − LL and P. Sh.

strictly.[3] These observations are commonly used as a base to determine the target correction in the surgical treatment of sagittal malalignment.

Another radiological parameter that emerged recently to analyze the spinal alignment in the sagittal plane is the pelvic shift (P. Sh.) (see **Fig. 2**), which describes the posterior offset of the pelvis with respect to the heels.[15] This parameter is especially useful to characterize the compensatory mechanisms adopted by patients with alignment disorders in order to regain a sustainable balancing.

Sagittal Imbalance and Compensatory Mechanisms

When pathologic changes to the alignment of single segments or longer regions occur, the human body may react with a compensatory mechanism to counterbalance it, or with a combination of different mechanisms. Typical degenerative changes that may induce compensation are the loss of LL (even on 1 or 2 levels due to degenerative disc disease), and the increase of kyphosis in the thoracic spine.[16,17] It is thought that the aim of compensatory mechanisms is to reduce the energy expenditure in standing and during daily activities. Indeed, an imbalanced posture requires a significant constant activation of the trunk muscles in order to counterbalance the weight of the upper body, which generates a moment with respect the feet due to its forward inclination.[3]

One of the first compensatory mechanisms that frequently occur also in asymptomatic elderly subjects is the retroversion of the pelvis,[18,19] which corresponds to a decrease of SS and an increase of PT (**Fig. 3**). In addition, single lumbar segments may exhibit hyperextension or retrolisthesis, thus creating a risk of stenosis of the spinal canal.[19,20] Another compensatory strategy detectable, especially in younger subjects having a good spine flexibility, is the reduction of TK, which combined with the loss of LL results in a relatively flat sagittal profile of the spine.[18] More severe cases show a flexion of the knees, which induces additional energy expenditure due to the recruitment of the thigh muscles and may generate anomalies in the gait pattern.[21]

The combined effect of these compensatory strategies can be effectively assessed by measuring P. Sh., which increases if the pelvis is retroverted and/or knees are flexed. Indeed, in several cases in which a loss of LL does not lead to an increased SVA (eg, due to pelvic retroversion), a gain of P. Sh. is still detectable[15,22] (compensated imbalanced spine). Whereas P. Sh. is therefore an indicator of the amount of the compensatory mechanisms, SVA is better suited to assess the part of the imbalance, which cannot be compensated and thus directly provokes functional impairments to the patient (imbalanced spine).

IMAGING PROTOCOLS

The radiological evaluation of the spinal alignment is commonly conducted by means of planar radiographs. The evaluation of most parameters (eg, PI, PT, LL, TK, SVA) can be performed on

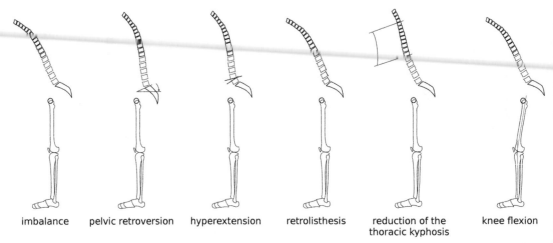

| imbalance | pelvic retroversion | hyperextension | retrolisthesis | reduction of the thoracic kyphosis | knee flexion |

Fig. 3. The most common compensatory mechanisms. Starting from an imbalanced condition (left), an improved alignment can be gained by (from left to right): pelvic retroversion, hyperextension, retrolisthesis, reduction of the TK, flexion of the knees. A combination of 2 or more of these mechanisms is frequently observed in clinical cases.

sagittal projections, including the thoracolumbar spine and the proximal femur, whereas the assessment of knee flexion and P. Sh. requires a lateral scan of the entire body. Patients having suspect degenerative scoliosis additionally require the acquisition of an anteroposterior projection. It is mandatory that all radiographic projections are captured in a free-standing, natural position, in order to avoid artifacts in posture-dependent parameters (eg, PT, SVA). To maximize the visualization quality and limit the superimposition of the arms and the spine, patients are usually asked to flex elbows and wrists and touch the supraclavicular fossa with the fingers.[23]

The recent introduction of the EOS Imaging System (EOS Imaging, Paris, France) had a remarkable impact on the clinical evaluation of the spinal alignment.[24–26] The EOS system allows for the simultaneous acquisition of whole-body biplanar projections with a radiation dose significantly lower than that of a single lumbar radiograph projection, with increased dynamic range and comparable image quality. Its use pioneered an extensive series of radiological studies in which the alignment of the entire body was evaluated in patients suffering from several abnormalities (reviewed in Ref.[27]).

As mentioned above, MR imaging provides excellent contrast within soft tissues, such as intervertebral disc and ligaments, and is therefore widely used for the diagnosis of spinal disorders related with such tissues. Indeed, one of the most commonly used scores to grade intervertebral disc degeneration, the Pfirrmann scale, is based on T2-weighted MR images.[28] This imaging modality is capable of clearly identifying

dehydrated discs, which appear dark in contrast to bright discs having high water content.[1] MR imaging also excels for the morphologic characterization of discs and surrounding structures. As a matter of fact, endplate lesions such as Schmorl nodes and the so-called Modic changes (which highlight inflammation processes as well as edema and bone marrow disorders), are investigated best by means of MR imaging scans.[29] Stenosis of the spinal canal[30] and arthrosis of the facet joints[31] can also be diagnosed. However, despite its excellence for the visualization of spinal tissues, MR imaging needs to be performed in a horizontal position (supine or prone posture) and therefore does not allow for a characterization of the spinopelvic alignment.[32] A few upright MR imaging scanners are indeed commercially available, but currently suffer from a limited image quality due to the low intensity of the magnetic field as well as high costs, which restrict their general availability.[32]

MR imaging may have specific relevance in distinguishing the spinal disorders initiating the degenerative cascade from those originating from compensatory mechanisms, which may be reversible and left untreated.[3] For example, in some patients having a reduced LL compensated by a reduced TK, after fixation and realignment of the lumbar spine, the thoracic compensation may disappear because it is not needed any more to restore an equilibrated condition. However, in more severe cases, a compensatory mechanism may structure itself into a proper degenerative disorder, therefore also requiring surgical treatment. Because of the qualities of MR imaging discussed above, an in-depth analysis of MR imaging scans may provide more useful than planar radiographs in distinguishing the reversible compensations from those needing treatment.

IMAGING FINDINGS: REPRESENTATIVE CLINICAL CASE

A 75-year-old male patient suffering from suspect spinal stenosis was referred to a spine surgeon and subsequently subjected to lumbar MR imaging scanning, which highlighted extensive degenerative changes in the entire lumbosacral spine (**Fig. 4**). Degenerative disc disease, discal protrusions, as well as osteophytosis were evident. In particular, foraminal stenosis was detected at L4-L5, whereas a transforaminal disc herniation was diagnosed at L3-L4. A subsequent CT scan (see **Fig. 4**) confirmed the severe degenerative changes detected by MR imaging and revealed in addition an extensive vacuum phenomenon in all lumbar intervertebral discs. It should be noted that both medical reports of the MR imaging and CT scans included mention of retrolistheses at L1-L2, L2-L3, and L3-L4, which

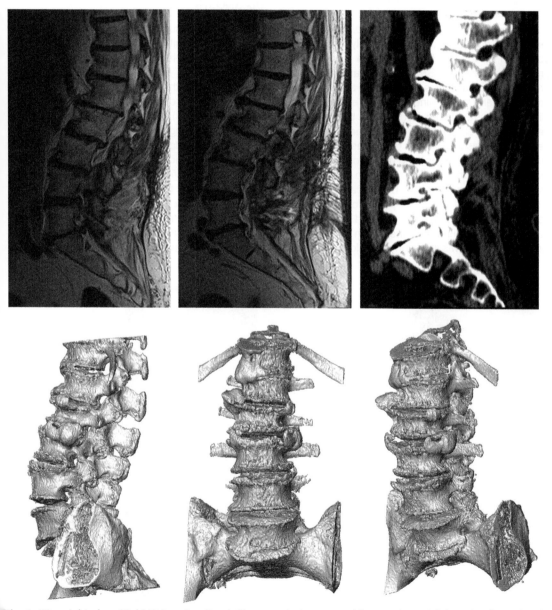

Fig. 4. T2-weighted sagittal MR imaging (*top left*), computed tomographic scans (*top right*), and 3-dimensional reconstruction (*botttom*) of the representative clinical case before the surgical treatment. Degenerated discs, protrusions, osteophytosis, and vertebral retrolistheses are evident.

may have indicated a compensatory mechanism due to an alignment disorder in the sagittal plane, which was not further investigated.

Based on these reports and on the clinical examination, decompression of the spinal canal and of the neural foramen at L4-L5 with subsequent fixation by means of a riveted interspinous implant was performed. Furthermore, decompression and implantation of a soft interspinous spacer were conducted at L3-L4. Nevertheless, despite minor improvements, the patient continued to suffer from radicular disorders after the surgical treatment.

Biplanar radiographs acquired with the EOS system 1 year after the surgery revealed a significant spine misalignment in the sagittal plane (**Fig. 5**). In view of a PI of 39°, an exceedingly low LL (20° between L1 and L5, 30° between L4 and S1) was measured. The low SS (13°) indicated a pelvic retroversion, which was exploited as a compensatory mechanism combined with the evident retrolistheses to regain an acceptable balance and equilibrium. It should be noted that these phenomena would presumably lead to increased stress on the posterior structures[3] and reduction of the neural space and are therefore related to the radicular symptoms. Despite that full body scans were not available, an additional compensation by means of knee flexion would be presumed based on a qualitative analysis of the orientation of the proximal femurs. TK was in the physiologic range (46°).

In general, based on the analysis of the radiographic data in the standing posture, the patient would have benefited from a long lumbosacral fixation with reconstruction of an appropriate LL instead of the simple decompression followed by interspinous stabilization. Even if taken in the supine position, the MR imaging findings of retrolistheses should have directed the surgeon to perform an orthostatic analysis of the entire lumbosacral spine, including at least the proximal femurs for the assessment of the spinopelvic parameters.

DIAGNOSTIC CRITERIA

The planning of surgical treatment of degenerative disorders in adult patients requires the analysis of the spinal alignment on full standing radiographs (posteroanterior and laterolateral views), in combination with the most typical signs of the degenerative disease (disc dehydration, stenosis, osteophytes), which can be detected by means of MR imaging and/or other imaging modalities. In particular, compensatory mechanisms (pelvic retroversion, knee flexion, retrolisthesis) need to be identified for correct surgical planning. MR imaging may find an additional specific role in distinguishing the primary spinal disorders from those originating from compensatory mechanisms, which may be therefore treated or not depending on their clinical condition and structuring.

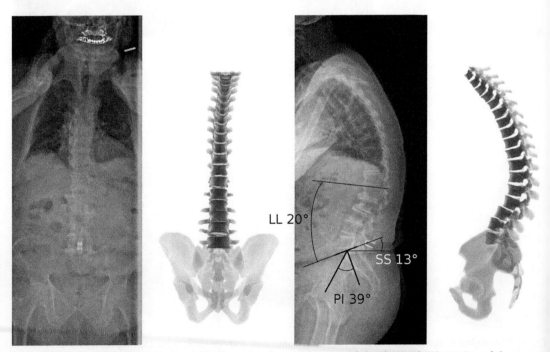

Fig. 5. Biplanar radiographic images and 3-dimensional reconstruction of the thoracolumbar spine of the representative patient after the surgical treatment, which still reveal a significant sagittal imbalance.

PEARLS, PITFALLS AND VARIANTS

- PI is the most important anatomic parameter (ie, not dependent on the posture), which contributes to the determination of the entire spine alignment.
- The analysis of single parameters describing imbalance may not be sufficient for a complete characterization of the alignment, as compensatory mechanisms may mask the disorder.
- Imaging in the standing posture is mandatory for the analysis of the alignment and therefore for an appropriate surgical planning.
- MR imaging is an excellent tool for the characterization of degenerative abnormalities and may be used to distinguish primary disorders from compensatory mechanisms.
- All planar radiographs must include the proximal femur (at least 10 cm).

WHAT THE REFERRING PHYSICIAN SHOULD KNOW

- The analysis of the spinopelvic alignment should always be performed when planning a surgery on a degenerated spine.
- Despite the wide availability of MR imaging scanners, planar radiography is still the imaging modality of reference for the evaluation of degenerative disorders in adult patients.

SUMMARY

A correct alignment of the spine is fundamental to avoid or minimize pain, limit the muscular effort to keep the standing posture, and allow for a good spine function during daily activities. In the present article, the most important radiological parameters describing the physiologic and pathologic alignment of the spine have been discussed, with special reference to the sagittal plane. The fundamental role of the pelvis and its morphology has been highlighted as well as the necessity of images in the standing posture for a proper analysis of the alignment. As extensively discussed, limiting diagnostic imaging to single motion segments or to short regions of the spine should nowadays be considered clinically inadequate, whereas a comprehensive evaluation of the entire spinopelvic alignment should always be performed.

REFERENCES

1. Brayda-Bruno M, Tibiletti M, Ito K, et al. Advances in the diagnosis of degenerated lumbar discs and their possible clinical application. Eur Spine J 2014; 23(Suppl 3):S315–23.

2. Lotz JC, Haughton V, Boden SD, et al. New treatments and imaging strategies in degenerative disease of the intervertebral disks. Radiology 2012; 264(1):6–19.

3. Lafage V, Diebo BG, Schwab F. Sagittal spino-pelvic alignment: from theory to clinical application. Madrid: Editorial Medica Panamericana; 2015.

4. Duval-Beaupere G, Schmidt C, Cosson P. A Barycentremetric study of the sagittal shape of spine and pelvis: the conditions required for an economic standing position. Ann Biomed Eng 1992;20(4):451–62.

5. Roussouly P, Gollogly S, Berthonnaud E, et al. Classification of the normal variation in the sagittal alignment of the human lumbar spine and pelvis in the standing position. Spine (Phila Pa 1976) 2005; 30(3):346–53.

6. Weinberg DS, Morris WZ, Gebhart JJ, et al. Pelvic incidence: an anatomic investigation of 880 cadaveric specimens. Eur Spine J 2015. [Epub ahead of print].

7. Schlosser TP, Janssen MM, Vrtovec T, et al. Evolution of the ischio-iliac lordosis during natural growth and its relation with the pelvic incidence. Eur Spine J 2014;23(7):1433–41.

8. Vialle R, Levassor N, Rillardon L, et al. Radiographic analysis of the sagittal alignment and balance of the spine in asymptomatic subjects. J Bone Joint Surg Am 2005;87(2):260–7.

9. Mac-Thiong JM, Berthonnaud E, Dimar JR 2nd, et al. Sagittal alignment of the spine and pelvis during growth. Spine (Phila Pa 1976) 2004;29(15):1642–7.

10. Yukawa Y, Kato F, Suda K, et al. Age-related changes in osseous anatomy, alignment, and range of motion of the cervical spine. Part I: radiographic data from over 1,200 asymptomatic subjects. Eur Spine J 2012;21(8):1492–8.

11. Gore DR, Sepic SB, Gardner GM. Roentgenographic findings of the cervical spine in asymptomatic people. Spine (Phila Pa 1976) 1986; 11(6):521–4.

12. Jackson RP, McManus AC. Radiographic analysis of sagittal plane alignment and balance in standing volunteers and patients with low back pain matched for age, sex, and size. A prospective controlled clinical study. Spine (Phila Pa 1976) 1994;19(14): 1611–8.

13. Schwab F, Patel A, Ungar B, et al. Adult spinal deformity-postoperative standing imbalance: how much can you tolerate? An overview of key parameters in assessing alignment and planning corrective surgery. Spine (Phila Pa 1976) 2010; 35(25):2224–31.

14. Schwab FJ, Blondel B, Bess S, et al. Radiographical spinopelvic parameters and disability in the setting of adult spinal deformity: a prospective multicenter analysis. Spine (Phila Pa 1976) 2013; 38(13):E803–12.

15. Lafage V, Schwab F, Skalli W, et al. Standing balance and sagittal plane spinal deformity: analysis of spinopelvic and gravity line parameters. Spine (Phila Pa 1976) 2008;33(14):1572–8.

16. Gelb DE, Lenke LG, Bridwell KH, et al. An analysis of sagittal spinal alignment in 100 asymptomatic middle and older aged volunteers. Spine (Phila Pa 1976) 1995;20(12):1351–8.

17. Farcy JP, Schwab FJ. Management of flatback and related kyphotic decompensation syndromes. Spine (Phila Pa 1976) 1997;22(20):2452–7.

18. Barrey C, Jund J, Noseda O, et al. Sagittal balance of the pelvis-spine complex and lumbar degenerative diseases. A comparative study about 85 cases. Eur Spine J 2007;16(9):1459–67.

19. Jackson RP, Peterson MD, McManus AC, et al. Compensatory spinopelvic balance over the hip axis and better reliability in measuring lordosis to the pelvic radius on standing lateral radiographs of adult volunteers and patients. Spine (Phila Pa 1976) 1998;23(16):1750–67.

20. Barrey C, Roussouly P, Perrin G, et al. Sagittal balance disorders in severe degenerative spine. Can we identify the compensatory mechanisms? Eur Spine J 2011;20(Suppl 5):626–33.

21. Obeid I, Hauger O, Aunoble S, et al. Global analysis of sagittal spinal alignment in major deformities: correlation between lack of lumbar lordosis and flexion of the knee. Eur Spine J 2011;20(Suppl 5):681–5.

22. Schwab F, Lafage V, Boyce R, et al. Gravity line analysis in adult volunteers: age-related correlation with spinal parameters, pelvic parameters, and foot position. Spine (Phila Pa 1976) 2006;31(25):E959–67.

23. Horton WC, Brown CW, Bridwell KH, et al. Is there an optimal patient stance for obtaining a lateral 36" radiograph? A critical comparison of three techniques. Spine (Phila Pa 1976) 2005;30(4):427–33.

24. McKenna C, Wade R, Faria R, et al. EOS 2D/3D X-ray imaging system: a systematic review and economic evaluation. Health Technol Assess 2012; 16(14):1–188.

25. Ilharreborde B, Dubousset J, Le Huec JC. Use of EOS imaging for the assessment of scoliosis deformities: application to postoperative 3D quantitative analysis of the trunk. Eur Spine J 2014; 23(Suppl 4):S397–405.

26. Al-Aubaidi Z, Lebel D, Oudjhane K, et al. Three-dimensional imaging of the spine using the EOS system: is it reliable? A comparative study using computed tomography imaging. J Pediatr Orthop B 2013;22(5):409–12.

27. Wade R, Yang H, McKenna C, et al. A systematic review of the clinical effectiveness of EOS 2D/3D X-ray imaging system. Eur Spine J 2013;22(2): 296–304.

28. Pfirrmann CW, Metzdorf A, Zanetti M, et al. Magnetic resonance classification of lumbar intervertebral disc degeneration. Spine (Phila Pa 1976) 2001; 26(17):1873–8.

29. Adams A, Roche O, Mazumder A, et al. Imaging of degenerative lumbar intervertebral discs; linking anatomy, pathology and imaging. Postgrad Med J 2014;90(1067):511–9.

30. Lee S, Lee JW, Yeom JS, et al. A practical MRI grading system for lumbar foraminal stenosis. AJR Am J Roentgenol 2010;194(4):1095–8.

31. Kotsenas AL. Imaging of posterior element axial pain generators: facet joints, pedicles, spinous processes, sacroiliac joints, and transitional segments. Radiol Clin North Am 2012; 50(4):705–30.

32. Alyas F, Connell D, Saifuddin A. Upright positional MRI of the lumbar spine. Clin Radiol 2008;63(9): 1035–48.

Neuroimaging of Spinal Canal Stenosis

Peter Cowley, MBBS (Lon), BA Oxon, MRCP, FRCR

KEYWORDS

- Spinal stenosis • Central canal stenosis • Lateral stenosis • Foraminal stenosis
- Neurogenic intermittent claudication • Cauda equina compression
- Cervical spondylotic myelopathy

KEY POINTS

- Spinal stenosis is a broad term encompassing central, lateral, and foraminal narrowing and implies compromise of the neural structures passing through that space.
- Imaging of spinal stenosis is primarily with MR imaging; however, CT and CT myelography (CTM) are acceptable alternatives.
- There is often a mismatch between imaging and clinical findings; accurate and rigorous interpretation of the imaging is necessary for correct management decisions.
- Cross-sectional imaging is usually acquired in a supine neutral position that under-recognizes the dynamic and load-bearing functions of the spinal column.

INTRODUCTION

The deceptively simple term, *spinal stenosis*, is actually a complex and multifaceted concept that means different things to different people. The purely anatomic observation of central canal stenosis implies a pathophysiology that is poorly understood and a set of clinical syndromes that correlate only loosely with the degree of stenosis. The ideal imaging modality that perfectly reflects the clinical presentation and predicts the future course of the pathophysiology is far from achieved, and as such it is essential for health care professionals to understand the limitations, the scope, and the potential of neuroimaging in the context of spinal stenosis.

Anatomically, spinal stenosis can be divided into cervical, thoracic, and lumbar forms because of variations in incidence, presentation, and management. The most common form is lumber canal stenosis, where neurogenic intermittent claudication (NIC) and radiculopathy dominate the clinical picture. Next is cervical canal stenosis with

associated myelopathy plus/minus radiculopathy. Thoracic canal stenosis is much rarer (at least as a result of degenerative/spondylotic pathoetiology) and also presents with myelopathy plus/minus radicular symptoms.

This article reviews

1. The congenital and degenerative circumstances underlying the physical narrowing of the spinal canal (including the central canal, the lateral recesses, and the neural foramina)
2. The pathophysiology of the clinical syndromes associated with spinal stenosis (ie, myelopathy, NIC, and radiculopathy)
3. Assessment of the strengths and weaknesses of the different imaging strategies, with an emphasis on MR imaging
4. Critical review of the different observational signs and objective criteria that have been proposed in the neuroimaging literature so far
5. Review of the application of upright scanning and axial loading in the diagnostic lexicon

The author has nothing to disclose.
National Hospital for Neurology and Neurosurgery, Neuroimaging Analysis Centre, UCLH, 3rd Floor, 8-11 Queen Square, London WC1N 3AR, UK
E-mail address: peter.cowley@nhs.net

Magn Reson Imaging Clin N Am 24 (2016) 523–539
http://dx.doi.org/10.1016/j.mric.2016.04.009

6. Assessment of the potential impact of advanced imaging strategies, such as diffusion tensor imaging

The primary substrate of spinal stenosis considered in this review is spondylosis; other acquired processes, such as neoplastic, traumatic, infective, and inflammatory pathologies leading to a secondary compressive effect on the spinal cord or cauda equine, are not specifically discussed in this review; however, there is an obvious crossover of understanding and imaging technique.

LUMBAR SPINAL STENOSIS

The North American Spine Society 2011 revised guidelines[1] provide the following definition:

Degenerative lumbar spinal stenosis describes a condition in which there is diminished space available for the neural and vascular elements in the lumbar spine secondary to degenerative changes in the spinal canal. When symptomatic, this causes a variable clinical syndrome of gluteal and/or lower extremity pain and/or fatigue, which may occur with or without back pain. Symptomatic lumbar spinal stenosis has certain characteristic provocative and palliative features. Provocative features include upright exercise, such as walking or positionally induced neurogenic claudication. Palliative features commonly include symptomatic relief with forward flexion, sitting, and/or recumbency.

Epidemiology/Prevalence

The initial description of mechanical compression of the cauda equine is attributed to Verbiest[6] from 1954; 60 years later, the incidence and natural history of the condition remain poorly documented. The Framingham Study data have been used by Kalichman and colleagues[2] to establish the prevalence of lumbar central canal stenosis in a community population. They used anterior-posterior dimensions less than 12 mm for relative stenosis and less than 10 mm for absolute stenosis on CT imaging (Table 1).

The frequency of acquired absolute stenosis of less than 10 mm increased from 4% in patients under age 40 to 14.3% in those over 60 years of age.

In this study the presence of absolute stenosis was significantly associated with low back pain but not leg pain. There review of the literature found a prevalence ranging from 1.7% to 13.1%.

The Japanese Wakayama Spine Study,[3] a population-based study of more than 1000 people, found a prevalence of symptomatic lumbar spinal stenosis of approximately 10%.

Table 1 The Framingham Study		
Framingham Study	Relative: Anterior-Posterior <12 mm	Absolute: Anterior-Posterior <10 mm
Congenital	4.7%	2.6%
Acquired	22.5%	7.3%

Data from Kalichman L, Cole R, Kim DH, et al. Spinal stenosis prevalence and association with symptoms: the Framingham study. Spine J 2009;9(7):545–50.

Given the wide variation in accepted criteria for defining lumbar spinal stenosis, it is unsurprising that there is considerable variation in the reported incidence and prevalence of the condition.

NATURAL HISTORY

There is a conspicuous absence of good-quality longitudinal studies documenting the natural history of patients with symptomatic lumbar canal stenosis. The North American Spine Society issued a statement that in the absence of reliable evidence, it is likely that the natural history of patients with mild to moderate symptomatic degenerative stenosis is favorable in one-third to one-half of patients. In patients with mild to moderate symptomatic stenosis, rapid or catastrophic neurologic decline is a rare phenomenon. There is no reliable evidence to define the natural history of clinically or radiologically severe stenosis.[1]

Congenital/Developmental Stenosis

Primary stenosis is uncommon, occurring in only 9% of cases. Congenital malformations include the following:

- Incomplete vertebral arch closure (spinal dysraphism)
- Segmentation failure
- Achondroplasia
- Osteopetrosis

Developmental flaws include the following:

- Early vertebral arch ossification
- Shortened pedicles
- Thoracolumbar kyphosis
- Apical vertebral wedging
- Anterior vertebral beaking (Morquio syndrome)
- Osseous exostosis

Acquired Stenosis

The most important structures underlying degenerative lumbar stenosis are the intervertebral disks, the facet joints, and the ligamentum flavum. The intervertebral disk may present with a herniation of the nucleus pulposus, a focal protrusion, or a broad-based bulge. Rarely does a disk bulge or protrusion cause a full-blown cauda equine syndrome in isolation. More often it is coupled with facet and flaval hypertrophy and/or congenital narrowing of the lumbar canal. Other features that may contribute are facet joint synovial cysts, facet and vertebral body osteophytes, and epidural lipomatosis. An important contributory pathology is spondylolisthesis, which, in the absence of pars defects, is strongly associated with lumbar canal stenosis.[4]

Systemic processes that may be involved in secondary stenosis include Paget disease, fluorosis, acromegaly, neoplasm, and ankylosing spondylitis.

CLINICAL PRESENTATION OF LUMBAR SPINAL STENOSIS

The diagnosis of lumbar spinal stenosis may be considered in older patients presenting with a history of gluteal or lower extremity symptoms exacerbated by walking or standing which improves or resolves with sitting or bending forward. Patients whose pain is not made worse with walking have a low likelihood of stenosis.[1]

There may be relative relief of symptoms on walking up an incline due to flexion of the lower spine. Saddle anesthesia and bladder disturbance are present in approximately 10% of cases. Fixed radicular symptoms of neuropathic pain and dysfunction may coexist due to lateral recess or foraminal stenosis.

The hallmark of central canal stenosis is the bilateral and ill-defined distribution with claudicant variation.

Presentation of intermittent leg pain and discomfort, usually during walking, shows sometimes subtle differences between the 2 pathologies of neurogenic claudication and peripheral arterial claudication. In both, walking becomes impossible but only in neurogenic claudication is stooping or sitting necessary to alleviate the symptoms. Likewise, claudication appears in both cases during walking whereas cycling is more associated by arterial disease. With advanced neurogenic claudication, descending stairs becomes impossible, forcing patients to walk downstairs backwards to adopt a forward flexed position; going upstairs is usually ok, in contrast to arterial pathologies in which all stair walking is difficult.[5]

Pathophysiology of Neurogenic Intermittent Claudication

The first description by Verbiest[6] postulated direct mechanical compression of the nerve roots in the generation of pain and dysfunction. Many experts believe that the positional and temporal presentation of the syndrome strongly suggests that dynamic factors, such as compression loading and postural change in the size of the canal, are crucial. The timescale of the relief on sitting and resting also suggests a vascular mediated process. Jinkins[7] has shown that enhancement indicating blood-nerve barrier breakdown is often present in lumbar canal stenosis. Furthermore, it occurs more readily due to outflow obstruction and venous engorgement than for inflow obstruction and arterial mediated ischemia.[8,9] Olmarker and colleagues[10] demonstrated that the capillaries and venules of the nerve root could be occluded by mild compression of approximately 30 mm Hg to 40 mm Hg. Takahashi and colleagues[11] found that the epidural pressure is only 15 mm Hg to 18 mm Hg during lumbar flexion in in lumbar canal stenosis patients but reaches 80 mm Hg to 100 mm Hg during lumbar extension. Ikawa and colleagues[12] have demonstrated ectopic firing and nerve dysfunction due to venous stasis in rat model. Additional observations by Sato and Kikuchi include the importance of 2 or more zones of stenosis, which significantly increas the chance of having NIC symptoms compared with a single-level stenosis.[13]

Inflammatory exudates, cerebrospinal fluid pressure changes and flow disturbance, endoneurial edema, and increased endoneurial compartment pressure have all been implicated in the pathogenesis of the nerve dysfunction and the clinical syndrome. Work by Morishita and colleagues[14] has emphasized the role of the neural foramen in generating nerve dysfunction.

The balance of evidence seems to suggest that the pathophysiology of NIC involves multifactorial pathways in which venous congestion plays an important role and identification of all levels of stenosis, including lateral recess and neural foramina as well as central canal, is essential.

Imaging Modality Recommendations for Lumbar Canal Stenosis

The North American Spine Society guidelines[1] state the following:

In patients with history and physical examination findings consistent with degenerative lumbar spinal stenosis, MR imaging is suggested as the most appropriate, noninvasive test to confirm the presence of anatomic narrowing of the spinal canal or the presence of nerve root impingement.

If MR imaging is either contraindicated or inconclusive, CTM is suggested as the most appropriate test to confirm the presence of anatomic narrowing of the spinal canal or the presence of nerve root impingement.

If MR imaging and CTM are contraindicated, inconclusive, or inappropriate, CT is the preferred test to confirm the presence of anatomic narrowing of the spinal canal or the presence of nerve root impingement.

MR imaging or CT with axial loading is suggested as a useful adjunct to routine imaging in patients who have clinical signs and symptoms of lumbar spinal stenosis, a dural sac area of less than 110 mm^2 at 1 or more levels, and suspected but not verified central or lateral stenosis on routine unloaded MR imaging or CT.

Kent and colleagues[15] undertook a systematic meta-analysis assessing the accuracy of CT, MR imaging, and myelography in diagnosing patients with lumbar spinal stenosis: they identified 14/116 relevant studies with a reference standard other than another imaging test. The sensitivity of MR imaging in the diagnosis of adult spinal stenosis was 81% to 97%, sensitivity of CT was 70% to 100%, and sensitivity of myelography was 67% to 78%.

Numerous more recent studies have demonstrated the approximate equivalence of MR imaging versus CTM for the diagnosis of lumbar spinal stenosis. Modic and colleagues[16] found the accuracy of MR imaging to be 82%, CT/CTM 83%, and myelography 71%, with respect to surgical findings at 151 examined levels. The concordance between MR imaging and CT/CTM was 86.8%. Schnebel and colleagues[17] retrospectively found 96.6% correlation between MR imaging and CTM.

The technical advances of MR imaging and CT technology have undoubtedly improved the quality and resolution of spinal imaging; it is difficult to quantify the relative changes brought about in both these modalities; however, there seems to be a general consensus that diagnostically, MR imaging is first line, with CT/CTM and conventional myelography satisfactory alternatives if required.

Standard MR imaging protocol

Sagittal T2-weighted (T2W) imaging with or without proton density images.

Turbo spin echo is preferred to gradient echo due to the susceptibility artefact causing overestimation of stenotic lesions.

Sagittal T1W imaging as standard.

Axial T2W imaging 3-mm to 5-mm slice thickness arranged perpendicular to longitudinal axis

at levels of interest. Correct alignment is clearly essential for anterior-posterior and dural sac area quantitative measurements.

Additional MR imaging sequences

High-resolution 3-D acquisition, for example, SPACE or CISS

Postcontrast with or without fat saturation

Diffusion tensor imaging and methods for axial loading

Quantitative Criteria for Lumbar Spinal Stenosis

Table 2 shows a simplified presentation of the findings from Steurer and colleagues,[37] who undertook a literature review of the quantitative radiologic signs used in the diagnosis of lumbar spinal stenosis.

Mamisch and colleagues[44] continued from this systematic review to perform a Delphi survey, polling 41 international experts in an attempt to gain a broad consensus on the qualitative and quantitative radiologic features of lumbar spinal stenosis. Results of the survey suggest that there are no broadly accepted quantitative criteria and only partially accepted qualitative criteria for a diagnosis of lumbar spinal stenosis. The latter include disk protrusion, lack of perineural intraforaminal fat, hypertrophic facet joint degeneration, absent fluid around the cauda equina, and hypertrophy of the ligamentum flavum. Cutoff values for the highest rated quantitative parameters given by the experts were 12 mm for the anteroposterior diameter of the osseous spinal canal (and midsagittal diameter of the dural sac), 3 mm for the diameter of the foramen, and 3 mm for the lateral recess height.

The multiplicity of quantitative measures that have been proposed over the past 3 decades is testament that none of them has proved satisfactory and it seems highly likely that a simple dimension definition of a complex pathology, such as spinal stenosis, is fundamentally flawed.

Degenerative Spondylolisthesis

First described by McNab[45] as "spondylolisthesis with an intact neural arch," vertebral displacement most commonly seen at L4/L5 is due to facet hypertrophy. It is common and affects 4% to 14%[46] of the elderly population, more frequently in women than men. Unlike isthmic spondylolisthesis, it is self-limiting and rarely reaches grade II; however, it can critically narrow the canal. Claudication, or more often radicular pain, is a symptoms of stenosis secondary to degenerative spondylolisthesis. Degenerative spondylolisthesis

Table 2
Signs used in the diagnosis of lumbar spinal stenosis

Central lumbar canal stenosis

Anterior-posterior diameter of canal/theca	Range: 10–15 mm (*and variously defined ratios of stenosis/normal*)[5,18–29]	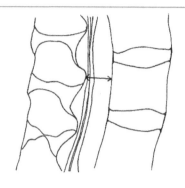
Cross-sectional area of canal/theca	Range: 100–130 mm² (*all modalities 75–145 mm², stenosis/normal ratios 0.62–0.73*)[20,23,30–34]	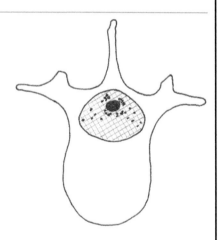
Ligamentous interfacet distance	Range: 10–13 mm (*10 mm at L2/L3, 13 mm at L5/S1*)[19,35,36]	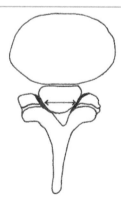

(continued on next page)

Table 2
(continued)

Transverse diameter of spinal canal	Range: 15–16 mm[18,23]	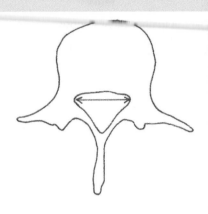
Lateral lumbar spinal stenosis		
Lateral recess height	≥5 mm: normal 3–5 mm: suggestive <3 mm: indicative[37–40]	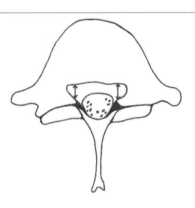
Lateral recess angle	<30°[40]	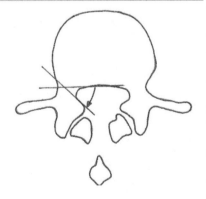
Lumbar foraminal stenosis	Range 3–4 mm Grade 0–3 focusing on obliteration of epidural fat and morphologic change of the nerve root[41–43]	—

normally affects a single level and thus is less likely to cause NIC. Central stenosis is rare in lytic spondylolisthesis but in some cases of L5/S1 displacement the posterior element can be pulled forward compressing the cauda against the body of S1.[47] More frequently, posterior disk bulging caused by the listhesis and loss of disk height can trap the nerve root in the foramen combined with facet hypertrophy to cause lateral recess stenosis. The osteofibrous callus present at the isthmic fracture level can occasionally hypertrophy to form Gill nodules[48] and compress the spinal canal.

Redundant Nerve Root and Sedimentation Signs

Redundant nerve roots of the cauda equina is a phrase first coined by Cressman and Pawl,[49,50] although the first descriptions are attributed to Verbiest. The entity characterized by elongated, enlarged, and tortuous nerve roots in the subarachnoid space adjacent to a level of lumbar spinal stenosis. The abnormality is seen above the level of the stenosis in 85%.[51] The presence of nerve thickening as well as elongation suggests a chronic reactive pathologic process repetitive traction and/or venous congestion. In the early stages, it seems likely that flexion/extension of the spine causes traction that pulls the roots through the stenosis, which then cannot slide back into position on returning the spine to a neutral position. The redundant nerve root sign is best appreciated in the sagittal plane on T2W sequences. It occurs in 34% to 42% of surgical candidates with NIC.[52] There was a tendency to increased age, worse clinical symptoms, and poorer postsurgical outcomes in the study by Min and colleagues.[52] Attempts to quantify the observational findings through measurement of the lengths of the redundant roots has not yet achieved a practical application. It remains a qualitative finding with interpretational subjectivity but is an important observation that should be looked for in all cases of central lumbar canal stenosis.

More recently Barz and colleagues[53] have described a nerve root sedimentation sign; it is considered positive if the roots of the cauda equina fail to sediment into the posterior half of the dural sac on either side of a stenotic lesion (on T2W axial images). This sign has been shown highly associated with high-grade lesions with dural sac area less than 80 mm^2; however, it is yet to be shown to add specificity (or sensitivity) in a general population.

It has long been noticed that the nerve roots at and either side of a stenosis demonstrate postgadolinium enhancement.[7] Kobayashi and colleagues[8] performed studies on dogs that applied circumferential pressure on the cauda equina. Histologic examination showed congestion and dilation in many of the intraradicular veins as well as inflammatory cell infiltration. The intraradicular edema caused by venous congestion and wallerian degeneration can also occur at sites that are not subject to mechanical compression. Enhanced MR imaging showed enhancement of the cauda equina at the stenosed region, demonstrating the presence of edema. This breakdown of the blood-nerve barrier not only is an important observation that has a role in improved specificity but also should not be mistaken for other pathologies.

DYNAMIC IMAGING

Imaging of the spine is routinely performed with the patient supine and in as relaxed a state as possible. The symptoms of spinal stenosis are commonly exacerbated by standing, walking, and extension. Imaging in extension versus neutral versus flexion and in an upright position or with axial loading applied have all been investigated to assess the relative effects on the spinal canal. Multiple studies have demonstrated a reduction in both dural sac area and midsagittal diameter on extension. Wei and colleagues[54] have attempted to quantify the dural sac area change versus angular rotation. Hansson and colleagues[55] showed that external load decreased the size of the spinal canal. Bulging of the ligamentum flavum contributed to between 50% and 85% of the spinal canal narrowing. It was concluded that the ligamentum flavum, not the disk, had the dominant role for load-induced narrowing of the lumbar spinal canal. Also, in the standing position, extension of the lumbar spine has the greater effect on canal narrowing compared with axial loading.

Greater changes in dural sac area with axial loading have been noted in older and in more symptomatic patients. There is reported correlation between stenosis present only on axially loaded patients and improved surgical outcomes.

Advanced Techniques

Eguchi and colleagues[56] performed a pilot study that elegantly demonstrated the ability of 3T systems to visualize lumbar nerve roots and structural abnormality, such as thinning, deviation, and interruption. Also the fractional anisotropy is decreased in the affected nerves in all their cases. The patients were highly selected for pure single-level degenerative radiculopathy with central canal stenosis and myelopathy excluded. Double-crush lesions have also been visualized with this technique (**Figs. 1–6**).[57]

CERVICAL STENOSIS

Cervical spondylosis is a common finding that increases with age. Degeneration of nucleus pulposus of the intervertebral disk leads to narrowing of the disk space, bulging of the annulus fibrosis, buckling of the ligamentum flavum, diskosteophyte bar formation, and hypertrophic osteoarthritic changes of the facet and uncovertebral joints. This cascade of degenerative processes may or may not result in cervical stenosis. As in the lumbar canal, cervical stenosis may refer to central, lateral, or foraminal narrowing. In contrast to the lumbar region, the clinically manifest lesions are dominated by foraminal stenosis, causing radicular symptoms, and central canal stenosis, causing myelopathy.

Clinical Presentations

Cervical pain may manifest locally or radiate to occiput, shoulder, scapular, and arm. There is variability with position may be associated with headache and interfere with sleep. The specific nerve roots involved demonstrate sensory and/or motor dysfunction. Pain, tingling, and dysesthesia are the most common presentations, with loss of fine motor skill, weakness, and muscle wasting also frequently present. The most commonly affected level is C5/C6 resulting in C6 radiculopathy; the next most commonly affected levels are C7 and C5.

First described by Stookey and Fleming in 1928,[58] compressive cervical spondylomyelopathy (CSM) has a more complex constellation of symptoms and signs. Patients with chronic mild CSM may be unaware of subtle changes in balance and fine motor dexterity.

Although culturally slightly specific, the Japanese Orthopaedic Association scale for spondylotic myelopathy[59] provides an excellent overview of the less subtle manifestations of cervical myelopathy (**Table 3**).

Detailed neurologic examination, including deep tendon reflexes and Hoffman, Romberg, and Babinski signs, are all important given the lack of diagnostic and prognostic accuracy that imaging has displayed.

Pathology of Cervical Spondylomyelopathy

It is widely acknowledged that both static and dynamic factors are implicated in the pathophysiology of CSM. Direct compression of the neural tissue is compounded by repetitive injury to cause secondary ischemia, inflammation, and apoptosis. The histologic hallmarks of the compressive myelomalacia are cystic cavitation and gliosis of the central grey matter and demyelination of the white matter long tracts. Wallerian degeneration extends caudally in the anterior horn cells and corticospinal tracts and rostral in the posterior columns and posterolateral tracts.

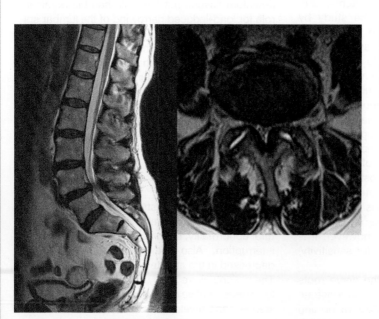

Fig. 1. Mild degenerative anterior listhesis at L4/L5 combines with posterior disk protrusion and thickening of the ligamentum flavum to result in bilateral L5 compressive radiculopathy.

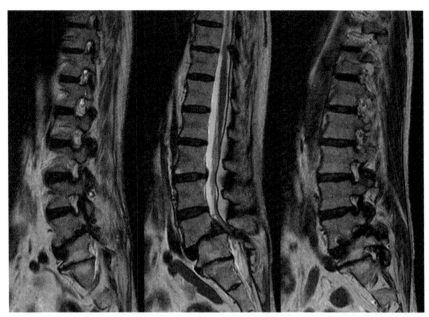

Fig. 2. Grade II spondylolisthesis with high-grade lumbar canal stenosis and bilateral L4 foraminal stenosis. The patient was unable to mobilize unaided and was complaining of sphincter disturbance.

Static and Dynamic Factors

The work of Morishita and colleagues[60] has shown that the constitutionally or developmentally narrow canal is an important factor in the etiology of CSM. Based on the midsagittal diameter of the canal at each segmental level, patients were classified as developmentally narrow less than 13 mm, normal 13 mm to 15 mm, and wide greater than 15 mm. They showed that developmentally narrow canals had a significantly increased frequency of cervical cord compression at all levels except C2/C3. Also they assessed the segmental angular motion in flexion and extension and found that those with developmentally narrow canals had significantly greater angular motion at C4/C5 to C6/C7 (although less at C3/C4), and this was associated with greater degenerative disk changes.

Several investigators have demonstrated decreased cross-sectional area of the cervical canal on both flexion and extension compared to the neutral position.[61–63] The greater decrease is seen in extension where buckling of the ligamentum flavum plays a major role.

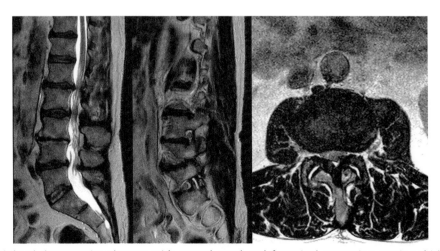

Fig. 3. Multilevel degenerative changes with central canal and foraminal narrowing causing thickened and serpiginous roots of the cauda equine: the redundant root sign.

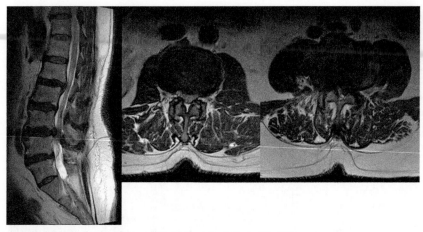

Fig. 4. Two-level lumbar canal stenosis is more likely associated with NIC.

Ossification of the posterior longitudinal ligament (OPLL) has been implicated in as many as 25% of cases of CSM in American and Japanese populations. The prevalence of OPLL is reported as 2 to 3 times higher in the Japanese and Asian populations than in the white population and is considerably more common in men, increasing with age. The pathoetiology of OPLL is multifactorial and strongly associated with diffuse idiopathic skeletal hyperostosis. It is also associated with ankylosing spondylitis and other spondyloarthropathies.[64]

Ossification of the ligamentum flavum is more commonly seen in the thoracic spine in Asian populations but may extend to the cervical region and combine with OPLL to cause canal stenosis and compressive myelopathy.

Imaging

MR imaging is the mainstay of cervical imaging, allowing excellent visualization of the soft tissue structures, good evaluation of canal dimensions and cross-sectional area of the cervical cord, and good sensitivity of any signal change present within the cord. Sagittal T2W and T1W imaging plus selected stacks of axial T2W images with or without T1W images are acquired as standard. Short tau inversion recovery images (STIR) may be added for additional sensitivity for bony and intramedullary lesions. For degenerative disk-osteophyte bars and ligamentous abnormality, turbo spin-echo T2W images have better clarity than gradient-echo T2W images; however, T2*W images may be more sensitive for intramedullary

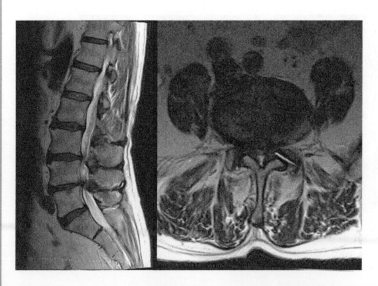

Fig. 5. Two-level stenosis secondary to slender disk protrusions combining with facet and flaval hypertrophy. Redundant root sign evident.

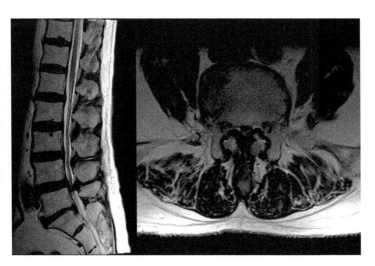

Fig. 6. Constitutionally narrow lumbar canal combines with ligamentum flavum hypertrophy or buckling to cause a high-grade canal stenosis.

hyperintensity. Diffusion tensor imaging has great promise to improve visualization of a functional correlate of both myelopathy and radiculopathy.

CT and CTM have advantages for assessment of OPLL and bony abnormalities and are useful alternatives when MR imaging is contraindicated. MR images consistently overestimate the degree of canal stenosis compared with CT and CTM.[65]

Specificity

Multiple studies have shown canal stenosis and cervical cord compression in asymptomatic patients. The prevalence increases with age and has been recorded at rates between 7% and 10% in patients over 60.[66] Conversely the severity of clinical presentation in patients with CSM has

Table 3
Japanese Orthopaedic Association scale for spondylotic myelopathy

Motor	Upper extremity	Unable to eat with spoon or chopsticks	0
		Possible to eat with spoon not chopsticks	1
		Possible to eat with chopsticks—but not adequate	2
		Possible to eat with chopsticks but awkward	3
		Normal	4
	Lower extremity	Impossible to walk	0
		Need a cane or aid on flat ground	1
		Need a cane or aid on stairs	2
		Possible to walk without a cane or aid but slow	3
		Normal	4
Sensory	Upper extremity	Apparent sensory loss	0
		Minimal sensory loss	1
		Normal	2
	Lower extremity	Apparent sensory loss	0
		Minimal sensory loss	1
		Normal	2
	Trunk	Apparent sensory loss	0
		Minimal sensory loss	1
		Normal	2
Sphincter	Bladder function	Complete retention	0
		Severe disturbance	1
		Mild disturbance	2
		Normal	3
TOTAL			17

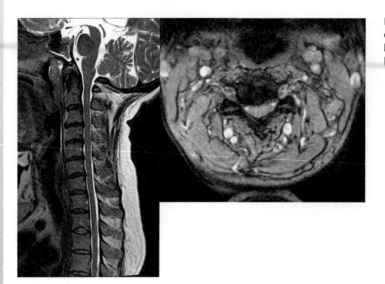

Fig. 7. A constitutionally narrow canal markedly increases the probability of developing cervical spondylotic myelopathy.

been found to correlate well with degree of canal narrowing.

Signal change within the cord remains a crucial observation with subtle ill-defined T2W hyperintensity likely representing reversible edema whereas bright well-defined T2W hyperintensity more likely is fixed gliosis/cystic necrosis/demyelination. T1W hypointensity almost certainly represents irreversible myelomalacia.

High-field systems now have the capability of acquiring diffusion tensor imaging, which allows mapping of the fractional anisotropy in the cord.

Reductions in fractional anisotropy have consistently been shown in canal stenosis and cervical cord compression. The clinical severity of CSM (inversely) correlates well with fractional anisotropy and postsurgical prognosis (**Figs. 7–14**).

THORACIC SPINAL STENOSIS

Degenerative thoracic stenosis occurs much less commonly than cervical or lumbar stenosis; this is likely due to the structural support of the rib cage and the relative reduced movement. When

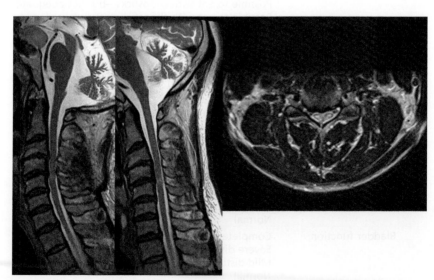

Fig. 8. Flexion extension sagittal T2W acquisitions reveal the exacerbation of the cervical stenosis in extension. Chronic myelopathic signal change already established.

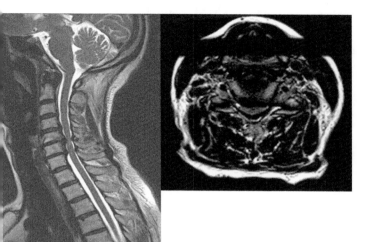

Fig. 9. C5/C6 and C6/C7 are the 2 most commonly affected levels for both compressive radicular and myelopathic lesions.

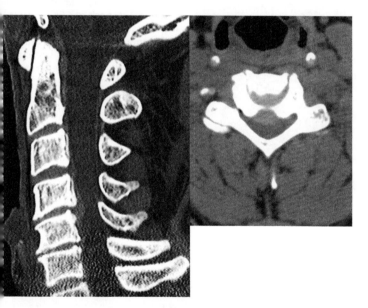

Fig. 10. Unenhanced CT with careful windowing provides reasonable visualization of disk and ligamentous as well as bony encroachment on the spinal canal.

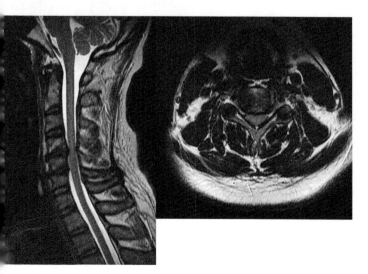

Fig. 11. Subtle diffuse signal change in the cord is more likely to represent reversible oedema compared with bright well-defined signal change with volume loss, which is more likely irreversible myelomalacia.

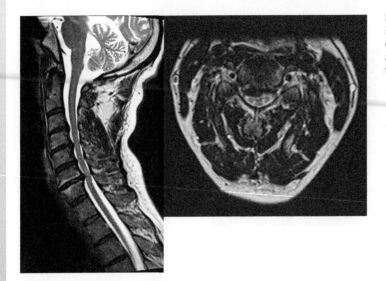

Fig. 12. The snake-eye appearance is associated with anterior horn cystic necrosis and venous infarction and is an unfavorable prognostic factor.

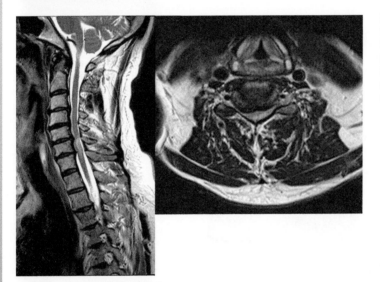

Fig. 13. Central, lateral, and foraminal stenosis at C5/C6, resulting in radicular and myelopathic symptoms. The cord signal change represents a mixture of cystic necrosis, wallerian degeneration, and edema.

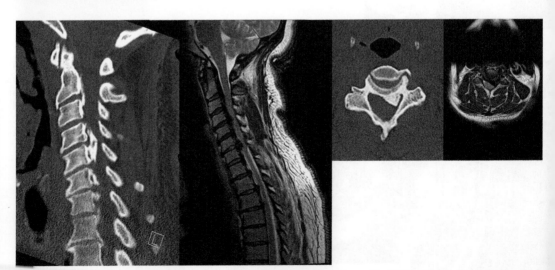

Fig. 14. OPLL is a multifactorial condition, which has a strong association with CSM. It is more frequently seen in Asian and elderly patients, and it is independently associated with diffuse idiopathic skeletal hyperostosis, ossification of the ligamentum flavum, and inflammatory spondyloarthropathies. CT and MR imaging are both required for assessment and management.

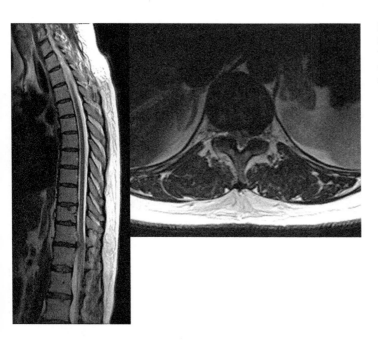

Fig. 15. The rarer thoracic spinal stenosis more often occurs in the lower thoracic region and results from combined anterior and posterolateral degenerative change.

it does occur, it is most frequently seen in the lower thoracic levels (T8–T12), possibly because of greater movement. The clinical presentation is that of myelopathy and/or radiculopathy and relates specifically to the level of the pathology. Disk-osteophyte bars and facet joint and ligamentum flavum hypertrophy remain the basic substrate, frequently combining with developmentally narrow canal to result in thoracic stenosis and neural compromise. Epidural lipomatosis and ossification of the ligamentum flavum are rare pathologies that may contribute to or be the sole cause of the stenosis (Fig. 15).

SUMMARY

MR imaging is first-line investigation of spinal stenosis. The site, extent, and number of stenotic lesions may be demonstrated with great resolution and clarity. Standard MR imaging sequences are unable, however, to visualize the dynamic changes that occur in the spine on loading and movement. Furthermore, they are largely unable to detect the subtle histopathologic changes that occur as a result of compression, repetitive strain, venous congestion, ischemia, and inflammatory processes. Additional imaging techniques, such as axial loading devices, upright scanning, flexion extension views, postgadolinium, and diffusion tensor imaging, have all shown insight into the specificity gap of conventional MR imaging and promise additional utility in the clinical setting.

REFERENCES

1. NASS revised 2011 guidelines for diagnosis and treatment of degenerative lumbar stenosis.
2. Kalichman L, Cole R, Kim DH, et al. Spinal stenosis prevalence and association with symptoms: the Framingham Study. Spine J 2009;9(7):545–50.
3. Ishimoto Y, Yoshimura N, Muraki S, et al. Prevalence of symptomatic lumbar spinal stenosis and its association with physical performance in a population-based cohort in Japan: the Wakayama Spine Study. Osteoarthritis Cartilage 2012;20(10):1103–8.
4. Herkowitz HN, Kurz LT. Degenerative lumbar spondylolisthesis with spinal stenosis. A prospective study comparing decompression with decompression and intertransverse process arthrodesis. J Bone Joint Surg Am 1991;73:802–8.
5. Szpalski M, Gunzburg R. Lumbar spinal stenosis in the elderly: an overview. Eur Spine J 2003; 12(Suppl 2):S170–5.
6. Verbiest H. A radicular syndrome from developmental narrowing of the lumbar vertebral canal. J Bone Joint Surg Br 1954;36-B(2):230–7.
7. Jinkins JR. Gd-DTPA enhanced MR of the lumbar spinal canal in patients with claudication. J Comput Assist Tomogr 1993;17(4):555–62.
8. Kobayashi S, Uchida K, Takeno K, et al. Imaging of cauda equina edema in lumbar canal stenosis by using gadolinium-enhanced MR imaging: experimental constriction injury. AJNR Am J Neuroradiol 2006;27(2):346–53.
9. Kobayashi S, Uchida K, Takeno K, et al. Pathophysiology, diagnosis and treatment of intermittent

claudication in patients with lumbar canal stenosis. World J Orthop 2014;5(2):134–45.

10. Ölmarker K, Rydevik R, Holm S. Edema formation in spinal nerve roots induced by experimental, graded compression. An experimental study on the pig cauda equina with special reference to differences in effects between rapid and slow onset of compression. Spine (Phila Pa 1976) 1989;14:569–73.

11. Takahashi K, Kagechika K, Takino T, et al. Changes in epidural pressure during walking in patients with lumbar spinal stenosis. Spine (Phila Pa 1976) 1995;20:2746–9.

12. Ikawa M, Atsuta Y, Tsunekawa H. Ectopic firing due to artificial venous stasis in rat lumbar spinal canal stenosis model: a possible pathogenesis of neurogenic intermittent claudication. Spine (Phila Pa 1976) 2005;30(21):2393–7.

13. Sato K, Kikuchi S. Clinical analysis of two-level compression of the cauda equina and the nerve roots in lumbar spinal canal stenosis. Spine (Phila Pa 1976) 1997;22(16):1898–903.

14. Morishita Y, Hida S, Naito M, et al. Measurement of the local pressure of the intervertebral foramen and the electrophysiological values of the epidural nerve roots in the vertebral foramen. Spine (Phila Pa 1976) 2006;31(26):3076–80.

15. Kent DL, Haynor DR, Larson EB, et al. Diagnosis of lumbar spinal stenosis in adults: a metaanalysis of the accuracy of CT, MR, and myelography. AJR Am J Roentgenol 1992;158(5):1135–44.

16. Modic MT, Masaryk T, Boumphrey F, et al. Lumbar herniated disk disease and canal stenosis: prospective evaluation by surface coil MR, CT, and myelography. AJR Am J Roentgenol 1986;147(4): 757–65.

17. Schnebel B, Kingston S, Watkins R, et al. Comparison of MRI to contrast CT in the diagnosis of spinal stenosis. Spine 1989;14(3):332–7.

18. Fukusaki M, Kobayashi I, Hara T, et al. Symptoms of spinal stenosis do not improve after epidural steroid injection. Clin J Pain 1998;14(2):148–51.

19. Koc Z, Ozcakir S, Sivrioglu K, et al. Effectiveness of physical therapy and epidural steroid injections in lumbar spinal stenosis. Spine (Phila Pa 1976) 2009;34(10):985–9.

20. Herzog RJ, Kaiser JA, Saal JA, et al. The importance of posterior epidural fat pad in lumbar central canal stenosis. Spine (Phila Pa 1976) 1991;16(6 Suppl): S227–33.

21. Bolender N, Schönström N, Spengler D. Role of computed tomography and myelography in the diagnosis of central spinal stenosis. J Bone Joint Surg Am 1985;67(2):240–6.

22. Haig AJ, Geisser ME, Tong HC, et al. Electromyographic and magnetic resonance imaging to predict lumbar stenosis, low-back pain, and no back symptoms. J Bone Joint Surg Am 2007;89(2):358–66.

23. Lee B, Kazam E, Newman A. Computed tomography of the spine and spinal cord. Radiology 1978; 128(1):95–102.

24. Ullrich C, Binet E, Sanecki M, et al. Quantitative assessment of the lumbar spinal canal by computed tomography. Radiology 1980;134(1):137–43.

25. Verbiest H. The significance and principles of computerized axial tomography in idiopathic developmental stenosis of the bony lumbar vertebral canal. Spine (Phila Pa 1976) 1979;4(4):369–78.

26. Airaksinen O, Herno A, Turunen V, et al. Surgical outcome of 438 patients treated surgically for lumbar spinal stenosis. Spine (Phila Pa 1976) 1997; 22(19):2278–82.

27. Herno A, Airaksinen O, Saari T. Computed tomography after laminectomy for lumbar spinal stenosis. Patients' pain patterns, walking capacity, and subjective disability had no correlation with computed tomography findings. Spine (Phila Pa 1976) 1994; 19(17):1975–8.

28. Jönsson B, Annertz M, Sjöberg C, et al. A prospective and consecutive study of surgically treated lumbar spinal stenosis. Part I: clinical features related to radiographic findings. Spine (Phila Pa 1976) 1997;22(24):2932–7.

29. Sortland O, Magnaes B, Hauge T. Functional myelography with metrizamide in the diagnosis of lumbar spinal stenosis. Acta Radiol Suppl 1977;355: 42–54.

30. Verbiest H. Neurogenic intermittent claudication in cases with absolute and relative stenosis of the lumbar vertebral canal (ASLC and RSLC), in cases with narrow lumbar intervertebral foramina, and in cases with both entities. Clin Neurosurg 1973;20: 204–14.

31. Hamanishi C, Matukura N, Fujita M, et al. Crosssectional area of the stenotic lumbar dural tube measured from the transverse views of magnetic resonance imaging. J Spinal Disord 1994;7(5): 388–93.

32. Mariconda M, Fava R, Gatto A, et al. Unilateral laminectomy for bilateral decompression of lumbar spinal stenosis: a prospective comparative study with conservatively treated patients. J Spinal Disord Tech 2002;15(1):39–46.

33. Laurencin C, Lipson S, Senatus P, et al. The stenosis ratio: a new tool for the diagnosis of degenerative spinal stenosis. Int J Surg Investig 1999;1(2): 127–31.

34. Schonstrom N, Bolender N, Spengler D. The pathomorphology of spinal stenosis as seen on CT scans of the lumbar spine. Spine (Phila Pa 1976) 1985; 10(9):806–11.

35. Schonstrom N, Willen J. Imaging lumbar spinal stenosis. Radiol Clin North Am 2001;39(1):31–53.

36. Wilmink J, Korte J, Penning L. Dimensions of the spinal canal in individuals symptomatic and

non-symptomatic for sciatica: a CT study. Neuroradiology 1988;30(6):547–50.

37. Steurer J, Roner S, Gnannt R, et al. Quantitative radiologic criteria for the diagnosis of lumbar spinal stenosis: a systematic literature review. BMC Musculoskelet Disord 2011;12:175.

38. Ciric I, Mikhael MA, Tarkington JA, et al. The lateral recess syndrome. A variant of spinal stenosis. J Neurosurg 1980;53(4):433–43.

39. Dincer F, Erzen C, Basgöze O, et al. Lateral recess syndrome and computed tomography. Turkish Neurosurg 1991;2:30–5.

40. Mikhael M, Ciric I, Tarkington J, et al. Neuroradiological evaluation of lateral recess syndrome. Radiology 1981;140(1):97–107.

41. Strojnik T. Measurement of the lateral recess angle as a possible alternative for evaluation of the lateral recess stenosis on a CT scan. Wien Klin Wochenschr 2001;113(Suppl 3):53–8.

42. Wildermuth S, Zanetti M, Duewell S, et al. Lumbar spine: quantitative and qualitative assessment of positional (upright flexion and extension) MR imaging and myelography. Radiology 1998;207:391–8.

43. Lee S, Lee JW, Yeom JS, et al. A practical MRI grading system for lumbar foraminal stenosis. AJR Am J Roentgenol 2010;194(4):1095–8.

44. Mamisch N, Brumann M, Hodler J, et al, Lumbar Spinal Stenosis Outcome Study Working Group Zurich. Radiologic criteria for the diagnosis of spinal stenosis: results of a Delphi survey. Radiology 2012; 264(1):174–9.

45. McNab I. Spondylolisthesis with an intact neural arch; the so-called pseudo-spondylolisthesis. J Bone Joint Surg Br 1950;32-B(3):325–33.

46. Kauppila LI, Eustace S, Kiel DP, et al. Degenerative displacement of lumbar vertebrae. A 25-year follow-up study in Framingham. Spine (Phila Pa 1976) 1998;23(17):1868–73 [discussion: 1873–4].

47. Wiltse LL, Rothman SLG. Lumbar and lumbosacral spondylolisthesis. In: Wiesel SW, Weinstein JN, Herkowitz H, et al, editors. The lumbar spin. Philadelphia: Saunders; 1996. p. 621–54.

48. Gill GG, Manning JG, White HL. Surgical treatment of spondylolisthesis without spine fusion; excision of the loose lamina with decompression of the nerve roots. J Bone Joint Surg Am 1955;37-A(3):493–520.

49. Cressman MR, Pawl RP. Serpentine myelographic defect caused by a redundant nerve root. Case report. J Neurosurg 1968;28(4):391–3.

50. Schizas C, Rienmuller A, Pierzchala K, et al. Redundant nerve root sign. EuroSpine Liverpool, UK; 2013.

51. Poureisa M, Daghighi MH, Eftekhari P, et al. Redundant nerve roots of the cauda equina in lumbar spinal canal stenosis, an MR study on 500 cases. Eur Spine J 2015;24(10):2315–20.

52. Min JH, Jang JS, Lee SH. Clinical significance of redundant nerve roots of the cauda equina in lumbar spinal stenosis. Clin Neurol Neurosurg 2008;110(1): 14–8.

53. Barz T, Melloh M, Staub LP, et al. Nerve root sedimentation sign: evaluation of a new radiological sign in lumbar spinal stenosis. Spine (Phila Pa 1976) 2010;35(8):892–7.

54. Wei F, Wang J, Zou J, et al. Effect of lumbar angular motion on central canal diameter: positional MRI study in 491 cases. Chin Med J 2010;123(11):1422–5.

55. Hansson T, Suzuki N, Hebelka H, et al. The narrowing of the lumbar spinal canal during loaded MRI: the effects of the disc and ligamentum flavum. Eur Spine J 2009;18(5):679–86.

56. Eguchi Y, Ohtori S, Orita S, et al. Quantitative evaluation and visualization of lumbar foraminal nerve root entrapment by using diffusion tensor imaging: preliminary results. AJNR Am J Neuroradiol 2011;32: 1824–9.

57. Kanamoto H, Eguchi Y, Suzuki M, et al. The diagnosis of double-crush lesion in the L5 lumbar nerve using diffusion tensor imaging. Spine J 2015;16(3): 315–21.

58. Stookey B, Fleming GWTH. Compression of the Spinal Cord due to Ventral Extradural Cervical Chondromas. (Arch. of Neur. and Psychiat., August, 1928.). Br J Psychiatry 1929;75(309):333.

59. Hukuda SMT, Ogata M, Schichikawa K, et al. Operations for cervical spondylotic myelopathy: a comparison of the results of anterior and posterior procedures. J Bone Joint Surg Br 1985;67B:609–15.

60. Morishita Y, Naito M, Hymanson H, et al. The relationship between the cervical spinal canal diameter and the pathological changes in the cervical spine. Eur Spine J 2009;18(6):877–83.

61. Chen IH, Vasavada A, Panjabi MM. Kinematics of the cervical spine canal: changes with sagittal plane loads. J Spinal Disord 1994;7(2):93–101.

62. Zhang L, Zeitoun D, Rangel A, et al. Preoperative evaluation of the cervical spondylotic myelopathy with flexion-extension magnetic resonance imaging: about a prospective study of fifty patients. Spine (Phila Pa 1976) 2011;36(17):E1134–9.

63. Muhle C, Weinert D, Falliner A, et al. Dynamic changes of the spinal canal in patients with cervical spondylosis at flexion and extension using magnetic resonance imaging. Invest Radiol 1998;33(8):444–9.

64. Saetia K, Cho D, Lee S, et al. Ossification of the posterior longitudinal ligament: a review. Neurosurg Focus 2011;30(3):E1.

65. Naganawa T, Miyamoto K, Ogura H, et al. Comparison of magnetic resonance imaging and computed tomogram-myelography for evaluation of cross sections of cervical spinal morphology. Spine (Phila Pa 1976) 2011;36(1):50–6.

66. Matsumoto M, Fujimura Y, Suzuki N, et al. MRI of cervical intervertebral discs in asymptomatic subjects. J Bone Joint Surg Br 1998;80(1):19–24.

Neuroimaging of the Traumatic Spine

Marcel Wolf, MD[a],*, Marc-André Weber, MD, MSc[b]

KEYWORDS

● Spine ● Trauma ● Spinal cord ● MR imaging ● Paraplegia

KEY POINTS

● In the absence of high-risk factors as defined, for instance, by the Canadian C-Spine Rule (CCR) in alert and stable trauma patients, no imaging is necessary at all.
● MR imaging is the imaging method of choice, when spinal cord injury, cord compression, or ligamentous injury is suspected, especially in obtunded patients.
● Direct injury of the spinal cord may result in ischemia, edema, and hemorrhage and MR imaging can detect these changes already in the hyperacute und acute stages.
● The incidence of posttraumatic syringomyelia increases with time period after the injury.

EPIDEMIOLOGY OF SPINAL TRAUMA

The rate of spinal trauma shows wide international variation. According to systemic reviews of international studies, the incidence and mortality of spinal column and spinal cord injuries are significantly higher in developing compared with developed countries.[1,2] For instance, in the United States, the incidence of traumatic spinal cord injury in 2010 was approximately 40 per million per year, or approximately 12,400 annually.[3] A bimodal age distribution is demonstrated in most studies, with a first peak in adolescents and young adults between 15 and 29 years of age and a second peak in adults older than 65 years of age. The mortality is significantly higher in older patients.[4] Spinal trauma is more common in men. In descending order, motor vehicle accidents, falls, violence, and sport accidents are the most common causes of spinal cord injuries.[5] The exposed localization and the higher degree of mobility between the head and torso predispose the cervical spine to injuries, in particular, the vertebrae around the craniocervical and cervicothoracal junction. The ribcage leads to more rigidity and stability of the thoracal spine compared with the thoracolumbar junction. Thus, spinal injuries are most often located in the cervical spine, followed by the thoracolumbar junction.[2]

INDICATIONS FOR IMAGING OF THE TRAUMATIC SPINE

In the United States, each year many trauma patients at risk for spine injury are treated in emergency departments, but only a small percentage of these patients have a spine fracture. To enhance the efficiency, sensitivity, and specificity of the utilization of radiologic examinations, and thus save resources, approved clinical decision tools or rules should be consulted to

Disclosure Statement: The authors have nothing to disclose.
[a] Neuroradiology, University Hospital Heidelberg, Im Neuenheimer Feld 400, Heidelberg D-69120, Germany;
[b] Diagnostic and Interventional Radiology, University Hospital Heidelberg, Im Neuenheimer Feld 110, Heidelberg D-69120, Germany
* Corresponding author.
E-mail address: marcel.wolf@med.uni-heidelberg.de

Magn Reson Imaging Clin N Am 24 (2016) 541–561
http://dx.doi.org/10.1016/j.mric.2016.04.004

Table 1
Low-risk criteria of National Emergency X-Radiography Utilization Study Low-Risk Criteria and Canadian C-Spine Rule

National Emergency X-Radiography Utilization Study Low-Risk Criteria	Low-Risk Canadian C-Spine Rule
Cervical spine radiography is indicated for patients with trauma unless they meet all of the following criteria: • No posterior midline cervical-spine tenderness • No evidence of intoxication or brain injury • Normal level of alertness • No focal neurologic deficit • No painful distracting injuries	No radiography is indicated, if any of the following 5 low-risk criteria is fulfilled: • Simple rear-end motor vehicle collision • Sitting position in emergency department • Ambulatory at any time • Delayed onset of neck pain • Absence of midline cervical tenderness And ability to rotate neck 45° left and right

determine if a radiologic examination is reasonable. These clinical decision rules consider variables from the patient history and examination or simple clinical tests, were derived from clinical research, and are defined as decision-making tools. The most established clinical decision rules for spinal imaging are the CCR[6–8] and the National Emergency X-Radiography Utilization Study Low-Risk Criteria (NLC)[9–11] (**Table 1**). By identifying high-risk criteria (**Box 1**), both clinical decision tools help if radiography is indicated as a screening method on alert (eg, score of 15 on the Glasgow Coma Scale) and stable trauma patients with mild or unspecific symptoms and low risk of spine injury. In the absence of high-risk

factors in alert and stable trauma patients, no imaging is necessary at all. When high risk-factors are identified in these patients, however, imaging is suggested.

A large prospective multicenter cohort study in 9 Canadian emergency departments, comparing the CCR and NLC in trauma patients in stable condition, showed that the CCR has a significantly higher sensitivity and specificity for cervical spine injury than the NLC, and that its consequent use would result in reduced rates of radiography.[12] Therefore, the CCR is visualized as standard operating procedure in **Fig. 1** and is used as reference at the authors' institution.

Box 1
Canadian C-Spine Rule high-risk criteria

High-risk criteria of CCR

Age greater than 65 years

Dangerous mechanism (ie, high-speed motor vehicle accident or fall from heights over 1m)

Paresthesia in extremities

Further high-risk criteria

Altered mental status

Multiple fractures

Drowning or diving accidents

Significant head or facial injury

Rigid spinal disease (ie, ankylosing spondylitis, diffuse idiopathic skeletal hyperostosis)

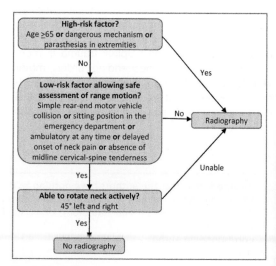

Fig. 1. The CCR.

In the acute phase of the injury period, flexion-extension radiography is not useful, because of muscle spasm, and dynamic fluoroscopy should not be used to evaluate for ligamentous injury in obtunded patients.[13]

In patients with high-risk criteria, multiple sites of trauma, correlating neurologic deficits or trauma mechanisms proposing an injury of the spine, imaging of the spine with computed tomography (CT) and if necessary, and not contraindicated, MR imaging is indicated. Among the advantages of CT is its widespread availability. Also, due to multidetector CT technology, CT needs a short time of image acquisition and CT has the potential of diagnostic evaluation of adjacent organs within the scanned body region. Moreover, CT yields an unsurpassed contrast of osseous structures. The radiation dose of a CT scan has to be considered, especially in young patients, and when scanning the pelvis and lumbar spine. Due to its superior soft tissue contrast, MR imaging is the method of choice for visualizing neural tissue, intervertebral disks,

and ligamentous structures. Nevertheless, an immediate MR imaging examination may be not possible in every emergency department, and the contraindications (eg, most cardiac pacemakers or other electrically stimulating implants and loose metallic objects), the long duration of the examination, and the potentially limited possibilities of patient monitoring during the MR imaging examination have to be taken into account. No contraindications assumed, an immediate MR imaging after spinal trauma is indicated when CT or neurologic symptoms suggest an injury of neural, or ligamentous structures and when an adequate neurologic examination cannot be performed, even when the CT scan turned out to be normal.

The American College of Radiology Appropriateness Criteria for Suspected Spine Trauma summarizes several conclusions.[13] No imaging should be performed in patients with positive low-risk criteria by NLC or CCR. In adults with high-risk criteria by NLC or CCR, multidetector CT (with multiplanar reformatting) is the

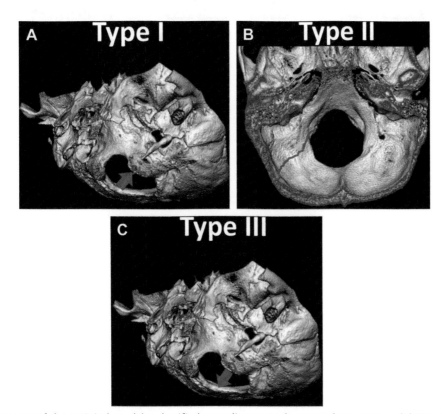

Fig. 2. Fractures of the occipital condyles classified according to Anderson and Montesano. (*A*) Type I, impacted fracture of the occipital condyle. (*B*) Type II, basilar skull fracture including an occipital condyle fracture. (*C*) Type III, displaced avulsion fracture on the occipital condyle.

recommended imaging method. Once a decision for imaging is made, the entire spine should be examined, considering the high incidence of noncontiguous multiple injuries. Thoracic and lumbar CT examinations can be derived from thoracic-abdomen-pelvis CT, instead of primary scanning of the spine. In children up to 14 years, radiography is the imaging method of choice: recommended views for cervical spine are anterior-posterior, lateral, and open mouth. Recommended views for thoracic and lumbar

spine are anterior-posterior and lateral. Because radiography has a limited diagnostic use in adults, it should be used primarily for resolving nondiagnostic CT scans due to motion artifacts. In the acute injury period, flexion-extension radiography is not useful, due to muscle spasm. MR imaging is the imaging method of choice, when spinal cord injury, cord compression, and/or ligamentous injury is suspected, especially in obtunded patients. Dynamic fluoroscopy should not be used for

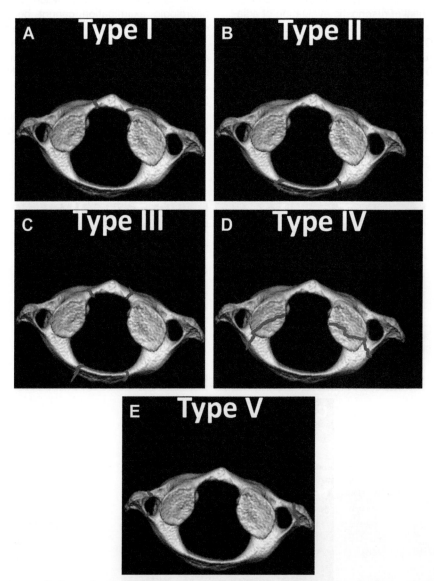

Fig. 2. Fractures of the axis classified according to Gehweiler. (A) Type I, fracture of the anterior arch. (B) Type II, fracture of the posterior arch. (C) Type III, combined fracture of anterior and posterior arch, so-called Jefferson fracture. (D) Type IV, fracture of lateral mass. (E) Type V, fracture of transverse process.

evaluation of ligamentous injury in obtunded patients.

RADIOLOGIC CLASSIFICATIONS OF SPINAL TRAUMA
Traditional Classification Schemes Based on Fracture Localization and Morphology

Traditional classification schemes of spinal fractures are exclusively based on description of the location and morphology of the fracture. Thus, CT or even plain radiography is sufficient for using these classifications.

Craniocervical junction
Occipital condyle fractures Anderson and Montesano[14] classified condyle fractures in 3 categories (**Fig. 2**): type I, impacted fracture of the occipital condyle; type II, basilar skull fracture, including an occipital condyle fracture; and type III,

displaced avulsion fracture on the occipital condyle. Types I and II are supposed to be stable, whereas type III is unstable, due to potentially associated tear of alar ligaments.

Atlas fractures The classification of fractures of the atlas, according to Gehweiler and colleagues,[15] differentiates 5 types: type I, fracture of the anterior arch; type II, fracture of the posterior arch; type III, combined fracture of anterior and posterior arch, so-called Jefferson fracture; type IV, fracture of lateral mass; and type V, fracture of transverse process (**Fig. 3**). Fractures of the atlas can be associated with injuries of the vertebral artery, in particular in type V fractures, indicating CT or MR angiography.

Odontoid fractures According to Anderson and d'Alonzo,[16] fractures of the odontoid process of

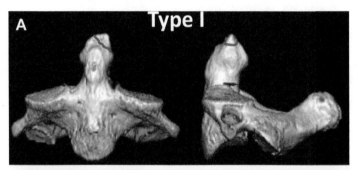
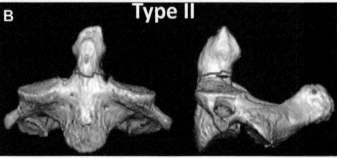
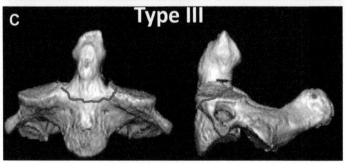

Fig. 4. Fractures of the odontoid classified according to Anderson and d'Alonzo. (*A*) Type I, avulsion of the odontoid tip. (*B*) Type II, fracture of odontoid body. (*C*) Type III, basilar fracture of the axis.

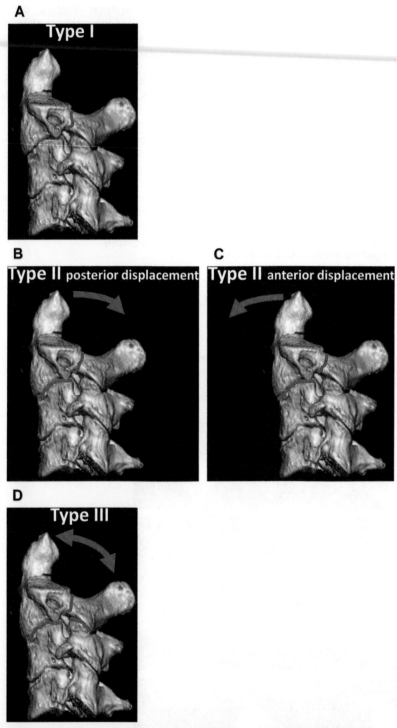

Fig. 5. Fractures of the axis classified according to Effendi. (*A*) Type I, isolated nondisplaced fracture. (*B, C*) Type II, traumatic spondylolisthesis with greater than 3 mm (*B*) posterior or (*C*) anterior displacement of C2 on C3 and disruption of C2/C3 disk. (*D*) Type III, traumatic spondylolisthesis with disruption of C2/C3 disk and disruption of facet joints.

the axis are classified in 3 types: type I, avulsion of the odontoid tip; type II, fracture of odontoid body; and type III, basilar fracture of the axis (**Fig. 4**). Although originally considered stable, the stability of type I fractures is discussed controversially, because of the avulsion of the apical odontoid ligament. Type II fractures are unstable, whereas most type III fractures are supposed to be stable.

Axis fractures Fractures of the axis with traumatic spondylolysis can be classified according to Effendi and colleagues[17] in 3 types: type I, isolated nondisplaced fracture; type II, traumatic spondylolisthesis with greater than or equal to 3-mm anterior displacement of C2 on C3 and disruption of C2/C3 disk; and type III, traumatic spondylolisthesis with disruption of C2/C3 disk and disruption of facet joints (**Fig. 5**). In fractures of the axis, the vertebral artery is at risk for injuries. In cases of axis fractures, an associated injury of the vertebral artery should be excluded by CT or MR angiography.

Thoracolumbar fractures Fractures of the thoracolumbar spine can be classified according to the 3-column model of Denis.[18] The anterior column includes the anterior longitudinal ligament and the anterior two-thirds of the vertebral body and intervertebral disk. The middle column includes the posterior third of the vertebral body and intervertebral disk and the posterior ligament. The posterior column includes spinous process, ligamentum flava, and the interspinous, supraspinous, and intertransverse ligaments (**Fig. 6**). Injuries of more than 1 column are unstable. Isolated injuries of the middle column are not possible. Usually, impaction fractures affect the anterior and middle column; flexion-distraction injuries affect the anterior and posterior column.

The most accepted and comprehensive classification of thoracal and lumbar spine fractures is based on Magerl[19] and was adopted by the AO Foundation. The trauma mechanism is classified as A (impaction), B (distraction), and C (rotation) (**Fig. 7**). To accommodate the variety and complexity of possible fractures, each of these 3 main categories can be categorized in subgroups. A0, minor, nonstructural fractures; A1, wedge-compression fractures; A2, split fractures; A3, incomplete burst fractures; A4, complete burst fractures; B1, posterior band disruption; B2, distraction of the posterior arch (Chance fracture); B3, hyperextension; C, multidirectional with translation, displacement,

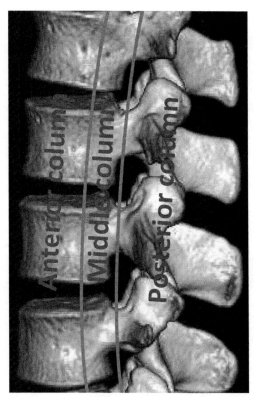

Fig. 6. 3-Column model according to Denis. Anterior column: anterior longitudinal ligament, anterior two-thirds of vertebral body, and intervertebral disk. Middle column: posterior third of vertebral body and intervertebral disk, and posterior ligament. Posterior column: spinous process, ligamentum flava and interspinous, supraspinous, and intertransverse ligaments.

or dislocation. Although established for thoracolumbar fractures, in clinical routine, this classification is often used for injuries of the cervical spine as well.

INNOVATIVE CLASSIFICATIONS, INCLUDING LIGAMENTOUS INTEGRITY AND NEUROLOGIC STATUS

Contrary to the traditional radiologic classification systems, merely considering the location and morphology of the fracture, the newer and more innovative classification systems of subaxial injury classification (SLICS)[20] and thoracolumbar injury classification and severity score (TLICS)[21] incorporate neurologic status and integrity of posterior ligamentous complex. Furthermore, based on a scoring system, a therapeutic recommendation toward conservative or surgical management

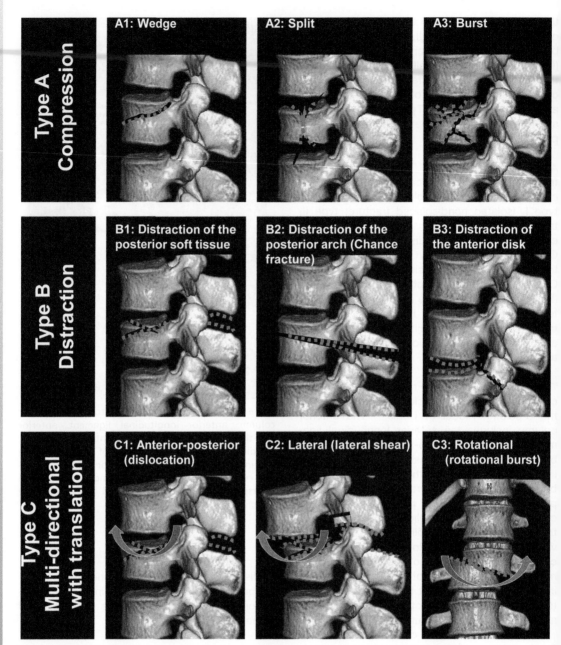

Fig. 7. Classification of thoracolumbar fractures according to Magerl and the AO Foundation.

is given by these more recent classification systems. Because TLICS (**Table 2**) and SLICS (**Table 3**) include evaluation of the posterior ligamentous complex, MR imaging found its way into these spine fracture classification systems. In particular, in the cervical spine, exclusive reliance on CT may lead to missed injuries that can be diagnosed by additional MR imaging.[22]

ADVANTAGE OF ADDITIONAL MR IMAGING IN SPINAL TRAUMA

Although CT has a higher resolution in visualizing osseous structures, MR imaging has a higher sensitivity in diagnosing occult fractures, so that additional MR imaging may change initial classification of acute traumatic spine injuries, based on CT.[23] MR imaging helps identifying

Table 2
Thoracolumbar injury classification and severity score

Morphology	0 No abnormality 1 Compression 2 Burst fracture 3 Rotation/translation 4 Distraction	Radiograph or CT
Posterior ligamentous complex	0 Intact 2 Suspected/indeterminate 3 Injured	MR imaging
Neurologic status	0 Intact 2 Root injury 2 Complete cord/conus medullaris injury 3 Incomplete cord/conus medullaris injury 3 Cauda equina syndrome	Physical examination
Score	$\leq$3 4 $\geq$5	Nonoperative treatment Consider conservative and surgical therapy Operative treatment

noncontiguous fractures (**Fig. 8**), discoligamentous injuries[24] (see **Fig. 8**; **Figs. 9** and **10**), and spinal hematoma (see **Fig. 10**); may change the initial CT-based classification according to the AO Foundation to higher types; and potentially may have an impact on decision making for treatment of traumatic spine fractures[25] (**Fig. 11**).

PATTERNS OF NEURAL INJURY OF THE SPINE

Due to various potential injury mechanisms and interindividual anatomic and pathologic preconditions, the spectrum of neural injuries of the spine and consequently of radiologic findings is wide, ranging from the lack of any pathologic imaging findings to the complete transection of the spinal cord.

Table 3
Subaxial injury classification

Morphology	0 No abnormality 1 Compression 2 Burst fracture 3 Distraction 4 Rotation/translation	Radiograph or CT
Posterior ligamentous complex	0 Intact 1 Indeterminate 2 Injured	MR imaging
Neurologic status	0 Intact 1 Root injury 2 Complete cord injury 3 Incomplete cord injury +1 Continuous cord compression (in setting of neurologic deficit)	Physical examination
Score	$\leq$3 4 $\geq$5	Nonoperative therapy Consider conservative and surgical treatment Operative treatment

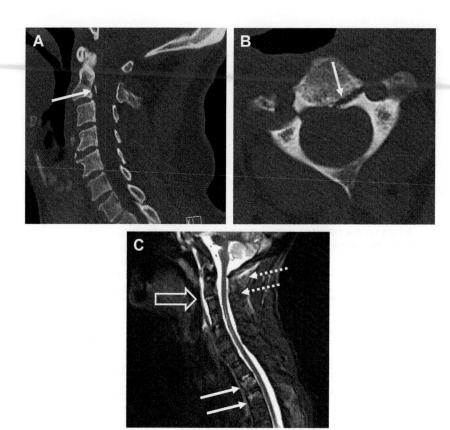

Fig. 8. Fracture of the axis, with rupture of the anterior longitudinal ligament and noncontiguous fractures of T2 and T3. CT ([*A*] sagittal and [*B*] axial) of the cervical spine showed nondislocated fractures (*arrow*) of the axis vertebra. (*C*) MR imaging with sagittal short tau inversion recovery revealed prevertebral hematoma (*open arrow*) ventral of C1 to C4, suggestive for rupture of the anterior longitudinal ligament, edema (*dotted arrows*) in the interspinal ligaments and the posterior atlantooccipital membrane, and noncontiguous impaction fractures of T2 and T3 (*small arrows*).

Spinal Cord Injury Without Radiographic Abnormality/Spinal Cord Injury Without Radiographic Evidence of Trauma

Symptomatic spinal cord injuries that show no correlate in radiographic or CT studies are referred to as spinal cord injury without radiographic abnormality or spinal cord injury without radiographic evidence of trauma, respectively. These conditions occur more frequently in children than in adults.[26] In most of these cases of a discrepancy of trauma-related neurologic symptoms and normal radiographs and/or CT scans, MR imaging shows injuries of the neural, or at least of the discoligamentous structures. The initial neurologic status correlates with the

MR imaging findings.[27,28] The recent meta-analyses showed that spinal MR imaging is of prognostic value in both children[29] and adults.[30] The rate of neurologic recovery is inversely correlated with the extent of cord involvement.

Spinal Cord Contusion: Intramedullary Edema and Hemorrhage

Direct mechanical injury of the spinal cord may result in local ischemia, edema, and hemorrhage. MR imaging is capable of detecting these changes already in the hyperacute und acute stages of spinal cord injury. Spinal cord edema may be accompanied by cord swelling and is hyperintense

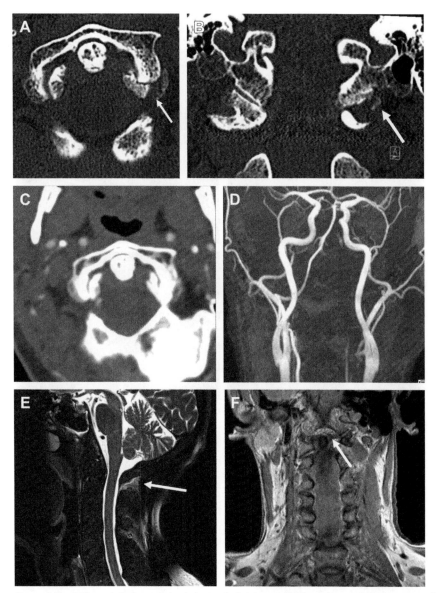

Fig. 9. Impaction of the left occipital condyle, injury of right vertebral artery, and ligamentous injuries. (*A*) Axial and (*B*) coronal CT images of an impaction of the left occipital condyle, with laterally displacement of a fragment (*arrow*). The suspected injury of the ipsilateral vertebral artery was diagnosed by (*C*) CT angiography and (*D*) MR angiography. (*E*) Sagittal fat-saturated T2-weighted images (revealed edema [*arrow*]) of the interspinal ligaments and posterior atlantooccipital membrane, indicating partial rupture. (*F*) Coronal proton density–weighted images showed continuity but increased signal intensity (*arrow*) in the left alar ligament, potentially indicating partial rupture.

on T2-weighted sequences and isointense to hypointense on T1-weighted images (**Fig. 12**). The signal intensity of spinal hematoma follows the typical MR aging appearance.[31,32] In the hyperacute stage, the oxygenated blood is isointense to hypointense on T1-weighted images and hyperintense on T2-weighted images. In the

following 2 days, during the acute phase, due to the deoxygenation of the hemorrhage, the signal intensity decreases on T1-weighted and T2-weighted images (**Fig. 13**). In the early subacute stage, from days 2 to 7, the transformation to methemoglobin results in an increase in T1 signal intensity and decrease in T2 signal intensity

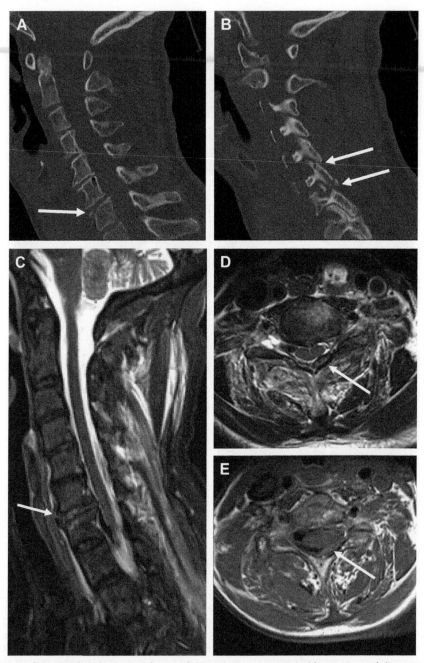

Fig. 10. Fracture of C7 vertebral body and facets of C6 and C7, accompanied by rupture of the anterior longitudinal ligament and an epidural hematoma. (*A*) Fracture of the anterior portion of the cranial endplate of C7 (*arrow* in [*A*]) and (*B*) fractures of the facets of C6 and C7 (*arrows* in [*B*]) are depicted on sagittal CT. (*C*) Sagittal short tau inversion recovery shows injury of the vertebral disk and disruption of the anterior longitudinal ligament C6/C7 (*arrow* in [*C*]). MR imaging also revealed epidural hematoma at the cervicothoracal junction (*arrow* in [*D*] axial T2-weighted image and [*E*] axial T1-weighted image).

(**Fig. 14**). Approximately 1 to 4 weeks after the hemorrhage, during the late subacute phase, the signal intensity is hyperintense on T1-weighted and T2-weighted images. More than 1 month after the initial hemorrhage during the chronic stage, the signal intensity gets isointense to hypointense on T1-weighted images and hypointense on T2-weighted images. T2* gradient-echo sequences

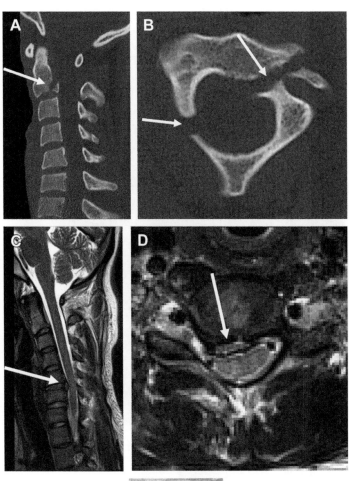

Fig. 11. Impact of additional MR imaging on decision making for treatment of spinal trauma. MR imaging helps identifying noncontiguous fractures and discoligamentous injuries and may potentially have an impact on decision making for treatment of traumatic spine fractures. (A) Sagittal and (B) axial CT images of fracture of the base and arch of the axis. Additional MR imaging revealed noncontiguous rupture of the disk 5/6 ([C] sagittal T2-weighted image), with right-sided disk extrusion and compression myelopathy ([D] axial T2-weighted image). The MR imaging–based diagnosis changed therapeutic decision making, leading to anterior diskectomy and fusion C5/C6, in addition to posterior fusion of C1 to C3, documented on (E) postoperative radiograph.

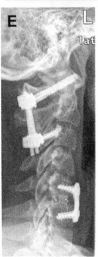

and susceptibility-weighted imaging (see **Fig. 14**) are most sensitive for detecting hemorrhages.[33] Intramedullary hemorrhages indicate a poorer prognosis compared with the sole presence of edema.[34,35]

Epidural and Subdural Hemorrhage

Spinal epidural (see **Figs. 10, 13,** and **14**) and subdural hemorrhages not only are induced by trauma, for instance iatrogenic or in accidents,

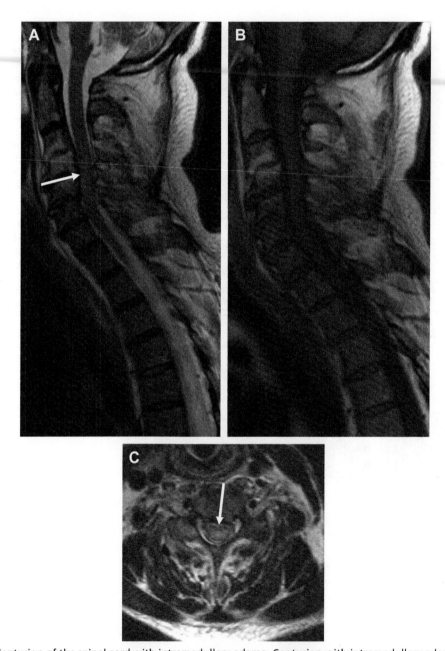

Fig. 12. Contusion of the spinal cord with intramedullary edema. Contusion with intramedullary edema (*arrow* in [*A*] and [*C*]) of the cervical spinal cord, with predisposing degeneration of the cervical spine, including spinal canal stenosis ([*A*] sagittal T2-weighted image, [*B*] sagittal T1-weighted image, and [*C*] axial T2-weighted image).

but also may rarely occur spontaneously in particular under anticoagulating medication.[36] Symptoms depend on the localization and extent of compression of the spinal cord. Early diagnosis and operative evacuation, if necessary, are essential for a favorable outcome. In certain cases, the localization of a spinal hemorrhage to the epidural or subdural compartment is difficult to assess. If a hemorrhage is located anteriorly in the spinal canal,

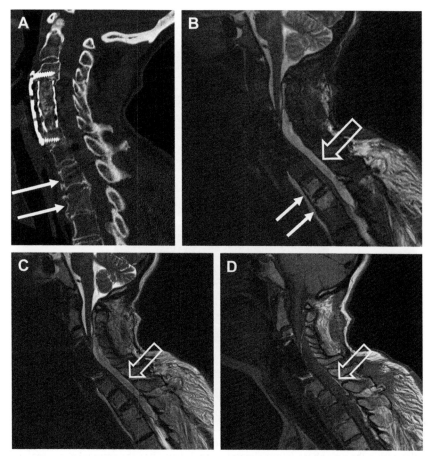

Fig. 13. Fracture of T1 and T2 with associated epidural hemorrhage. Fracture of T1 and T2 on sagittal CT (*arrows* in [*A*]). The corresponding bone marrow edema is visible on sagittal short tau inversion recovery (*arrows* [*B*]). (*D*) The T1 signal intensity of the epidural hematoma (*open arrow* [*B–D*]) is isointense or hypointense during the hyperacute (first 12 hours) and acute stage (12–48 hours). (*C*) The T2 signal intensity is hyperintense in the hyperintense stage and decreases during the acute stage.

the curtain sign may help in differentiating these 2 compartments.[37] Epidural hemorrhages may lift the dura from the bony spinal canal, except ventrally in the median line, where the dural sac is attached to the posterior longitudinal ligament by the Trolard membrane. Thus, the curtain sign is negative in spinal subdural hematomas.

Nerve Root Avulsion

Due to the high degree of mobility of the cervical spine, and the traction of the arms, traumatic nerve root avulsions are usually located cervicothoracally. Complete avulsions result in pseudomeningoceles, which are pathologic collections of cerebrospinal fluid. Pseudomeningoceles communicate with the physiologic cerebrospinal fluid spaces, but in contrast to the latter,

they are not covered by dura. The avulsion of nerve roots can be directly visualized by high-resolution T2-weighted sequences,[38] for instance, depending on the MR imaging manufacturer—constructive interference in steady state (CISS) or fast imaging employing steady-state acquisition (FIESTA) as well as sampling perfection with application optimized contrasts by using different flip angle evolutions (SPACE), CUBE, or volumetric isotropic TSE acquisition (VISTA)—whereas the posttraumatic pseudomeningoceles are generally visible on T2-weighted images with 3-mm to 5-mm slice thickness (**Fig. 15**).

Transection

Transections of the spinal cord (**Fig. 16**), partial or complete, are most often caused by luxation

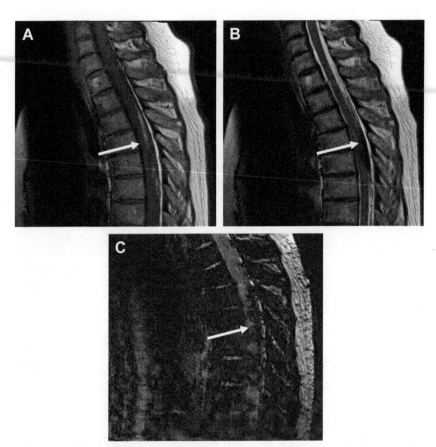

Fig. 14. Epidural hemorrhage in the thoracic spine. The signal intensity of spinal hematoma (*arrow*) is time-dependent. In the early subacute phase (approximately 1 to 7 days after the trauma) the signal intensity is predominantly (*A*) hyperintense on T1-weighted images and (*B*) hypointense on T2-weighted images. (*C*) Susceptibility-weighted imaging is most sensitive for detecting hemorrhage.

fractures, located in the thoracic spine, and result in a complete, or less frequently incomplete, paraplegia. The partial or complete discontinuity of the spinal cord can be visualized with MR imaging and is in the acute and subacute stage accompanied by edema and hemorrhage.

Myelomalacic Myelopathy

In the chronic stage after traumatic spinal cord injury, myelomalacic myelopathy may reside, showing a focal T2-hyperintense defect and often atrophy, caused by wallerian degeneration, in particular, caudal to the initial contusion.[39]

Posttraumatic Syringomyelia

After severe spinal cord injury, a posttraumatic syringomyelia (**Fig. 17**) may develop, which is a fusiform intramedullary cystic cavitation. Contrary to the central canal, a syringomyelia is not covered by ependyma. A syringomyelia must be differentiated from a hydromyelia, a pathologic dilatation of the central canal, and a ventriculus terminalis, a cavity filled with cerebrospinal fluid and located in the medullar conus. These 2 entities are both covered by ependyma. Potential clinical symptoms of a posttraumatic syringomyelia depend on the location and extent. Symptoms may be various and unspecific, including spasticity, neuropathic pain, loss of sensory and temperature sensation, motor loss, or hyperhidrosis. The pathogenesis of a posttraumatic syringomyelia is multifactorial, with compromised circulation of cerebrospinal fluid, caused by arachnopathic scarring, playing a crucial role. Posttraumatic syringomyelias originate most often at the location of the initial

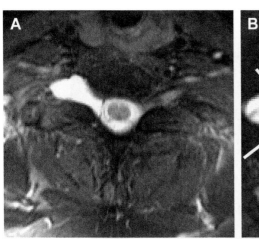
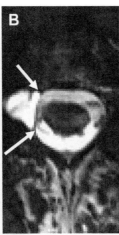
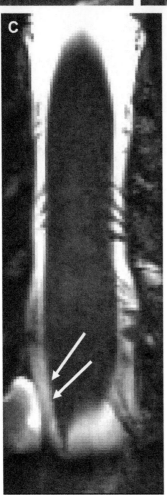

Fig. 15. Avulsion of cervical nerve rootlets. (*A*) The posttraumatic pseudomeningoceles are already visible on T2-weighted images with a slice thickness of 4.5 mm, whereas the proximal avulsion of the nerve rootlets (*arrows* in [*B*] and [*C*]) can be directly visualized on high-resolution T2-weighted sequences, like CISS with 0.75-mm slice thickness ([*B*] axial and [*C*] coronal multiplanar reconstructions of CISS).

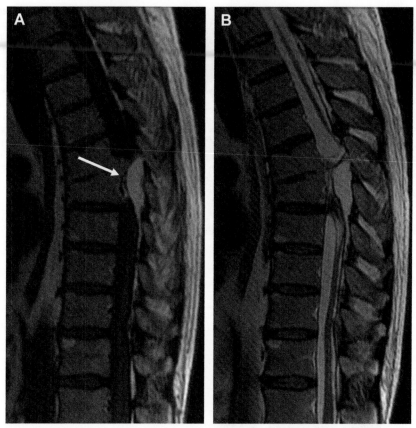

Fig. 16. Transection of the myelon. Sagittal (*A*) T1-weighted and (*B*) T2-weighted images in the chronic stage after spinal cord transsection. Note the atrophy of the spinal cord, due to wallerian degeneration. The arrow in (*A*) indicates a lipoma in location of the transection.

lesion but may ascend later, even years after the initial trauma, potentially worsening the neurologic status and elevating the level of the initial neurologic lesion.

EPIDEMIOLOGY OF POSTTRAUMATIC SYRINGOMYELIA

The incidence of posttraumatic syringomyelia varies in the literature and ranges from 3.5% to 4.3% in large collectives of paraplegic patients.[40,41] The incidence increases with time period of evaluation. For instance, more than 20 years after the injury, the incidence in paraplegic patients reaches approximately 21%.[42]

DIAGNOSIS OF POSTTRAUMATIC SYRINGOMYELIA

Because posttraumatic syringomyelia may develop or increase even years after the spinal

injury, spinal MR imaging is indicated when neurologic symptoms occur or worsen. Syringomyelia may also develop after meningitis, related to tumors, for instance ependymoma, or be associated with malformations, like Chiari malformation or Dandy- Walker malformation. To rule out neoplasms, in every newly diagnosed syringomyelia, contrast-enhanced MR imaging of the whole neural axis should be performed. High-resolution T2-weighted images, like CISS, may be helpful to detect arachnoid adhesions,[43] potentially facilitating planning surgical procedures. The disturbance of cerebrospinal fluid circulation can be detected with modern innovative MR imaging methods. With pulse- or ECG-gated phase contrast or steady state free precession sequences, the altered dynamics of cerebrospinal fluid flow can be detected and potentially quantified.[44–46]

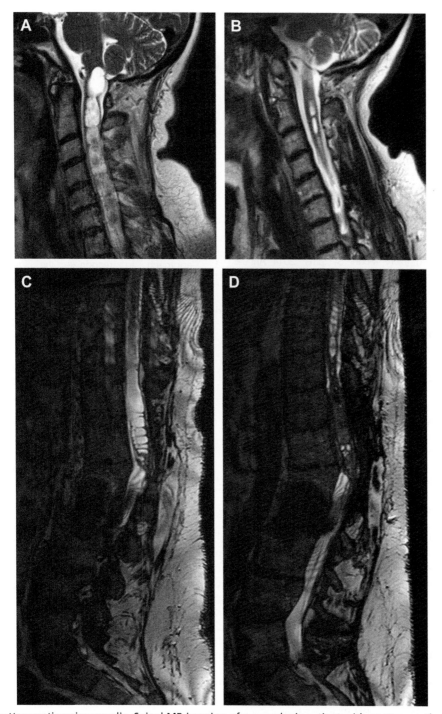

Fig. 17. Posttraumatic syringomyelia. Spinal MR imaging of a paraplegic patient with posttraumatic syringomyelia after burst fracture of L2. (*A*) and (*C*) show sagittal T2-weighted images of an extended syringomyelia ranging from the medulla oblongata to the medullar conus. (*B*) and (*D*) show sagittal T2-weighted images of the same patient after dorsal decompression, arachnolysis, and duraplasty. Surgery has led to a significant decreased extension of the syringomyelia.

REFERENCES

1. Chiu WT, Lin HC, Lam C, et al. Review paper: epidemiology of traumatic spinal cord injury; comparisons between developed and developing countries. Asia Pac J Public Health 2010;22(1):9–18.

2. van den Berg ME, Castellote JM, Mahillo-Fernandez I, et al. Incidence of spinal cord injury worldwide: a systematic review. Neuroepidemiology 2010;34(3):184–92.

3. DeVivo MJ. Epidemiology of traumatic spinal cord injury: trends and future implications. Spinal Cord 2012;50(5):365–72.

4. Fassett DR, Harrop JS, Maltenfort M, et al. Mortality rates in geriatric patients with spinal cord injuries. J Neurosurg Spine 2007;7(3):277–81.

5. NSCISC National Spinal cord Injury Statistical Center: Spinal Cord Injury Model Systems: 2014 Annual Report. 2015. 1-1-2016. Available at: https://www.nscisc.uab.edu/PublicDocuments/reports/pdf/2014%20NSCISC%20Annual%20Statistical%20Report%20Complete%20Public%20Version.pdf.

6. Canadian CT Head and C-Spine (CCC) Study Group. Canadian C-Spine Rule study for alert and stable trauma patients: I. Background and rationale. CJEM 2002;4(2):84–90.

7. Canadian CT Head and C-Spine (CCC) Study Group. Canadian C-Spine Rule study for alert and stable trauma patients: II. Study objectives and methodology. CJEM 2002;4(3):185–93.

8. Stiell IG, Wells GA, Vandemheen KL, et al. The Canadian C-spine rule for radiography in alert and stable trauma patients. JAMA 2001;286(15):1841–8.

9. Hoffman JR, Schriger DL, Mower W, et al. Low-risk criteria for cervical-spine radiography in blunt trauma: a prospective study. Ann Emerg Med 1992;21(12):1454–60.

10. Hoffman JR, Wolfson AB, Todd K, et al. Selective cervical spine radiography in blunt trauma: methodology of the National Emergency X-Radiography Utilization Study (NEXUS). Ann Emerg Med 1998;32(4):461–9.

11. Mahadevan S, Mower WR, Hoffman JR, et al. Interrater reliability of cervical spine injury criteria in patients with blunt trauma. Ann Emerg Med 1998;31(2):197–201.

12. Stiell IG, Clement CM, McKnight RD, et al. The Canadian C-spine rule versus the NEXUS low-risk criteria in patients with trauma. N Engl J Med 2003;349(26):2510–8.

13. Daffner RH, Weissman BN, Wippold FJI, et al. Expert Panels on Musculoskeletal and Neurologic Imaging. ACR Appropriateness Criteria® suspected spine trauma. American College of Radiology (ACR); 2012. p. 20. Available at: http://www.guideline.gov/content.aspx?id=37931.

14. Anderson PA, Montesano PX. Morphology and treatment of occipital condyle fractures. Spine (Phila Pa 1976) 1988;13(7):731–6.

15. Gehweiler JA, Duff DE, Martinez S, et al. Fractures of the atlas vertebra. Skeletal Radiol 1976;1:97–102.

16. Anderson LD, D'Alonzo RT. Fractures of the odontoid process of the axis. J Bone Joint Surg Am 1974;56(0):1663–74.

17. Effendi B, Roy D, Cornish B, et al. Fractures of the ring of the axis. A classification based on the analysis of 131 cases. J Bone Joint Surg Br 1981;63-B(3):319–27.

18. Denis F. The three column spine and its significance in the classification of acute thoracolumbar spinal injuries. Spine (Phila Pa 1976) 1983;8(8):817–31.

19. Magerl F, Aebi M, Gertzbein SD, et al. A comprehensive classification of thoracic and lumbar injuries. Eur Spine J 1994;3(4):184–201.

20. Vaccaro AR, Hulbert RJ, Patel AA, et al. The subaxial cervical spine injury classification system: a novel approach to recognize the importance of morphology, neurology, and integrity of the disco-ligamentous complex. Spine (Phila Pa 1976) 2007; 32(21):2365–74.

21. Vaccaro AR, Lehman RA Jr, Hurlbert RJ, et al. A new classification of thoracolumbar injuries: the importance of injury morphology, the integrity of the posterior ligamentous complex, and neurologic status. Spine (Phila Pa 1976) 2005;30(20):2325–33.

22. Schoenfeld AJ, Bono CM, McGuire KJ, et al. Computed tomography alone versus computed tomography and magnetic resonance imaging in the identification of occult injuries to the cervical spine: a meta-analysis. J Trauma 2010;68(1):109–13.

23. Winklhofer S, Thekkumthala-Sommer M, Schmidt D, et al. Magnetic resonance imaging frequently changes classification of acute traumatic thoracolumbar spine injuries. Skeletal Radiol 2013;42(6):779–86.

24. Choi SJ, Shin MJ, Kim SM, et al. Non-contiguous spinal injury in cervical spinal trauma: evaluation with cervical spine MRI. Korean J Radiol 2004;5(4): 219–24.

25. Pizones J, Izquierdo E, Alvarez P, et al. Impact of magnetic resonance imaging on decision making for thoracolumbar traumatic fracture diagnosis and treatment. Eur Spine J 2011;20(Suppl):3390–6.

26. Lee JH, Sung IY, Kang JY, et al. Characteristics of pediatric-onset spinal cord injury. Pediatr Int 2009; 51(2):254–7.

27. Mohanty SP, Bhat NS, Singh KA, et al. Cervical spinal cord injuries without radiographic evidence of trauma: a prospective study. Spinal Cord 2013; 51(11):815–8.

28. Sun LQ, Shen Y, Li YM. Quantitative magnetic resonance imaging analysis correlates with surgical outcome of cervical spinal cord injury without radiologic evidence of trauma. Spinal Cord 2014;52(7): 541–6.

29. Boese CK, Oppermann J, Siewe J, et al. Spinal cord injury without radiologic abnormality in children: a

systematic review and meta-analysis. J Trauma Acute Care Surg 2015;78(4):874–82.

30. Boese CK, Lechler P. Spinal cord injury without radiologic abnormalities in adults: a systematic review. J Trauma Acute Care Surg 2013;75(2):320–30.

31. Kidwell CS, Wintermark M. Imaging of intracranial haemorrhage. Lancet Neurol 2008;7(3):256–67.

32. Wasenko JJ, Lieberman KA, Rodziewicz GS, et al. Magnetic resonance imaging characteristics of hyperacute hemorrhage in the brain and spine. Clin Imaging 2002;26(5):330–7.

33. Wang M, Dai Y, Han Y, et al. Susceptibility weighted imaging in detecting hemorrhage in acute cervical spinal cord injury. Magn Reson Imaging 2011; 29(3):365–73.

34. Flanders AE, Spettell CM, Friedman DP, et al. The relationship between the functional abilities of patients with cervical spinal cord injury and the severity of damage revealed by MR imaging. AJNR Am J Neuroradiol 1999;20(5):926–34.

35. Mahmood NS, Kadavigere R, Avinash KR, et al. Magnetic resonance imaging in acute cervical spinal cord injury: a correlative study on spinal cord changes and 1 month motor recovery. Spinal Cord 2008;46(12):791–7.

36. Holtas S, Heiling M, Lonntoft M. Spontaneous spinal epidural hematoma: findings at MR imaging and clinical correlation. Radiology 1996;199(2):409–13.

37. Kuker W, Thiex R, Friese S, et al. Spinal subdural and epidural haematomas: diagnostic and therapeutic aspects in acute and subacute cases. Acta Neurochir (Wien) 2000;142(7):777–85.

38. Gasparotti R, Ferraresi S, Pinelli L, et al. Three-dimensional MR myelography of traumatic injuries of the brachial plexus. AJNR Am J Neuroradiol 1997;18(9):1733–42.

39. Falcone S, Quencer RM, Green BA, et al. Progressive posttraumatic myelomalacic myelopathy: imaging and clinical features. AJNR Am J Neuroradiol 1994;15(4):747–54.

40. el Masry WS, Biyani A. Incidence, management, and outcome of post-traumatic syringomyelia. In memory of Mr Bernard Williams. J Neurol Neurosurg Psychiatry 1996;60(2):141–6.

41. Schurch B, Wichmann W, Rossier AB. Post-traumatic syringomyelia (cystic myelopathy): a prospective study of 449 patients with spinal cord injury. J Neurol Neurosurg Psychiatry 1996;60(1):61–7.

42. Wang D, Bodley R, Sett P, et al. A clinical magnetic resonance imaging study of the traumatised spinal cord more than 20 years following injury. Paraplegia 1996;34(2):65–81.

43. Roser F, Ebner FH, Danz S, et al. Three-dimensional constructive interference in steady-state magnetic resonance imaging in syringomyelia: advantages over conventional imaging. J Neurosurg Spine 2008;8(5):429–35.

44. Bunck AC, Kroger JR, Juttner A, et al. Magnetic resonance 4D flow characteristics of cerebrospinal fluid at the craniocervical junction and the cervical spinal canal. Eur Radiol 2011;21(8): 1788–96.

45. Gottschalk A, Schmitz B, Mauer UM, et al. Dynamic visualization of arachnoid adhesions in a patient with idiopathic syringomyelia using high-resolution cine magnetic resonance imaging at 3T. J Magn Reson Imaging 2010;32(1):218–22.

46. Li AE, Wilkinson MD, McGrillen KM, et al. Clinical applications of cine balanced steady-state free precession MRI for the Evaluation of the Subarachnoid Spaces. Clin Neuroradiol 2015;25(4): 349–60.

Neuroimaging of Spinal Tumors

Zulejha Merhemic, MD, PhD[a],*, Tatjana Stosic-Opincal, MD, PhD[b],
Majda M. Thurnher, MD[c]

KEYWORDS

- Tumor • Spine • Intradural

KEY POINTS

- Magnetic resonance (MR) imaging is the method of choice for the detection and evaluation of intradural spinal lesions.
- There are numerous types of intradural-extramedullary masses, but meningioma and schwannoma are the most common tumors.
- Signal intensities, contrast enhancement pattern, and presence of cysts are key imaging findings in differentiation of spinal cord tumors.

Intradural spinal tumors are rare tumors with nonspecific clinical symptoms, usually occurring in the late stage of the disease, which results in delayed diagnosis. Back pain, radicular symptoms, slowly progressive neurologic deficits, or skeletal deformities, such as kyphoscoliosis, are commonly observed in children.

Intramedullary tumors comprise 20% to 30% of all primary intradural spinal tumors. The remaining 70% to 80% of primary intradural tumors are located in the intradural-extramedullary compartment.[1]

Magnetic resonance (MR) imaging is the method of choice for the detection and evaluation of intradural spinal lesions. The imaging protocol should include sagittal and axial T1-weighted and T2-weighted sequences, including contrast-enhanced T1-weighted sequences in the sagittal, axial, and coronal planes. Short time inversion recovery (STIR) should be added for the evaluation of intramedullary cord lesions as well as for the detection of bone abnormalities. Some advanced techniques, such as diffusion-weighted imaging and diffusion tensor imaging (DTI), have recently been described and are increasingly used in the evaluation of spinal lesions.[2]

DTI and fiber tractography are novel techniques with potential usefulness in preoperative diagnosis and postoperative follow-up of spinal cord tumors. These techniques provide more details about the white matter tracts in relation to space-occupying lesions, and thus, may be more sensitive than conventional MRI. Exploiting tractography in these cases has been helpful in predicting the nature of the lesion preoperatively and in planning the surgical intervention.[3]

Myelography and computed tomography (CT)-myelography are less frequently used for intradural spinal lesions. Angiography will be necessary to demonstrate the vascularization of hemangioblastomas (HBs) and presurgical interventions, such as the embolization of hypervascular lesions.[4]

Spinal PET/CT using fludeoxyglucose or 11(C) methionine has been used to evaluate intramedullary lesions, particularly for tumors with high-grade malignancy. Differentiation of tumors

The authors have nothing to disclose.
[a] Policlinic Sunce-Agram, University of Sarajevo, Trg medunarodnog prijateljstva 20, Sarajevo BiH-71000, Bosnia & Herzegovina; [b] General Hospital Euromedik, University of Belgrade, Visegradska 20, Belgrade 11000, Serbia; [c] Department of Biomedical Imaging and Image-Guided Therapy, Medical University Vienna, Waehringer Guertel 18-20, Vienna A-1090, Austria
* Corresponding author.
E-mail address: merhemic.zulejha@gmail.com

Magn Reson Imaging Clin N Am 24 (2016) 563–579
http://dx.doi.org/10.1016/j.mric.2016.04.007

with low-grade malignancy from non-neoplastic lesions may still prove challenging.[5]

Analysis of the cerebrospinal fluid (CSF) may help to decide among differential diagnoses with an inflammatory etiology.

INTRAMEDULLARY TUMORS
Ependymoma

Ependymoma is the most common primary spinal cord tumor in adults (60% of all primary spinal cord neoplasms), with 39 years of age the mean age of presentation. This is the second most common primary spinal cord tumor in children. Ependymoma is a slowly growing tumor originating from the wall of the ventricles or from ependyma lining the spinal cord central canal. There are 4 histologic ependymoma subtypes: cellular, myxopapillary, clear-cell, and tanycytic. The World Health Organization (WHO) currently classifies ependymomas into 3 grades: grade I tumors include myxopapillary ependymomas and subependymomas, grade II includes classic ependymomas, and grade III includes anaplastic ependymomas.[6] Although these grade classifications may be helpful in treatment decisions, the prognostic value is still controversial.

Ependymoma may be associated with neurofibromatosis type 2 (NF2). In NF2, most ependymomas are WHO grade II, and, rarely, WHO III (anaplastic ependymoma).

Cellular ependymoma are located mostly in the cervical and thoracic spinal cord, with a slight female predilection. They are well defined (may even be encapsulated masses), span up to 4 segments, and have cystic presentations in 50% to 90% of cases. Cysts usually have CSF intensity. The solid portion of the tumor is isointense or mildly hypointense on T1-weighted images (T1WI), hyperintense on T2-weighted images (T2WI) and STIR, and always enhances after contrast administration.[7]

The "cap sign" (hemosiderin on cranial or caudal margin) due to hemorrhage strongly suggests cord ependymoma. Syrinx is also a common finding (Fig. 1).

Myxopapillary ependymoma (MPE) is most commonly a tumor of the conus medullare or the filum terminale. It originates from ependymal cells of the filum terminale, and it is classified as a WHO grade I tumor. Ninety percent of all filum terminale tumors are myxopapillary ependymomas, with a male predilection. These tumors present with high-T2, iso or low-T1 signal intensity masses with strong but inhomogeneous enhancement (Fig. 2). Scalloping of the vertebral bodies, scoliosis, and enlargement of the neural foramina are

additional findings suggestive of myxopapillary ependymoma. Although MPEs are characterized as histologically benign, slow-growing tumors, some patients demonstrate local recurrence or even distant metastasis, more likely occurring in the pediatric population.[8]

Tanycytic ependymoma is a rare subtype of WHO grade II ependymoma. Histologically, these tumors have spindle cells arranged in a fascicular pattern, an absence of ependymal rosettes, and inconspicuous perivascular pseudorosettes.[9] A recently published meta-analysis of all described cases did not find any specific imaging finding. Most commonly, a solid mass with T1 hypointense or isointense signal and T2 hyperintensity, with or without a cystic component with an associated syringomyelic cavity, has been reported.[9]

The best outcomes for spinal ependymomas are achieved with total resection. More specifically, the classic grade II ependymomas may benefit most from aggressive resection, whereas myxopapillary grade I ependymomas did not have clear benefits from total resection.[10]

Astrocytoma

Astrocytoma is an intramedullary infiltrating mass present in 5% to 10% of all central nervous system (CNS) tumors. It is the most common neoplasm in children and the second most common in adults. Astrocytomas are composed of neoplastically transformed astrocytes, which vary from well differentiated to anaplastic. In almost 90% of cases, astrocytomas are low-grade neoplasms. An astrocytoma that extends along the entire length of the spinal cord is termed a "holocord" tumor. These are uncommon, and predominantly seen in children.

Fibrillary astrocytoma (WHO II) is usually seen in the cervical spine, whereas pilocytic astrocytoma (WHO I) is found mostly in the conus medullaris (Fig. 3). In 10% to 15% of these cases, high-grade astrocytoma also can occur, mostly anaplastic astrocytoma. The glioneuronal tumor with neuropil-like islands is a newly described variant of the anaplastic astrocytoma (WHO II or III).[11]

Several cases have been reported in the spinal cord, recently also with diffuse meningeal dissemination.[12] Glioblastomas in the spine are uncommon.

Astrocytomas are mostly solid masses extending to multiple vertebral levels. They can show areas of necrotic-cystic degeneration, can have a "cyst with a mural nodule" appearance, or can be completely solid (approximately 40% of the cases). The solid portion of the tumor is isointense or mildly hypointense on T1WI, hyperintense on T2WI and T2*GE,

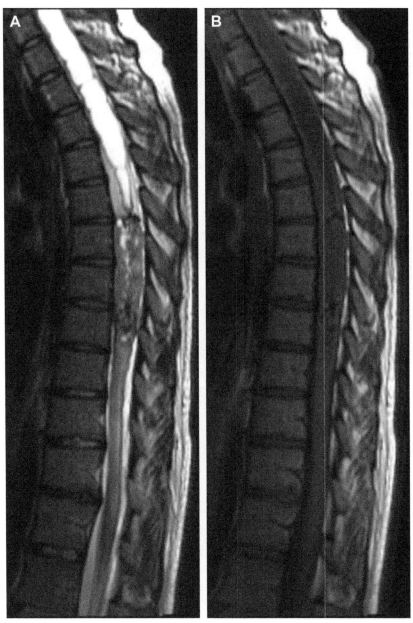

Fig. 1. Cellular ependymoma. Sagittal T2-weighted (*A*) and T1-weighted (*B*) MR images show an intramedullary mass extending from the T6 to the T8 level. Hemosiderin deposits are seen peripherally ("cap sign"), a common finding in ependymomas. In addition, multiple cyst formation is seen, as well as an associated syrinx in the upper thoracic and cervical cord.

and may show mild to moderate contrast enhancement. On DTI, long-tract fibers may be interrupted. The cystic part is usually moderately hyperintense to CSF on T2WI. Differentiation of neoplastic (enhancing wall) from non-neoplastic cysts (nonenhancing wall) is crucial for surgical planning.

Astrocytomas have an association with NF-1.[13] Based on one study on intramedullary tumors in NF-1, intramedullary spinal cord tumors associated with NF-1 tend to occur predominantly in male patients and are histopathologically likely to be an astrocytoma.[14]

Hemangioblastoma

HB of the CNS is a benign neoplasm that is classified as a WHO grade 1 tumor. It usually occurs in the cerebellum, brainstem, and spinal cord. HBs comprise 2% to 10% of all primary spinal cord tumors, and 60% to 75% of HBs are disseminated

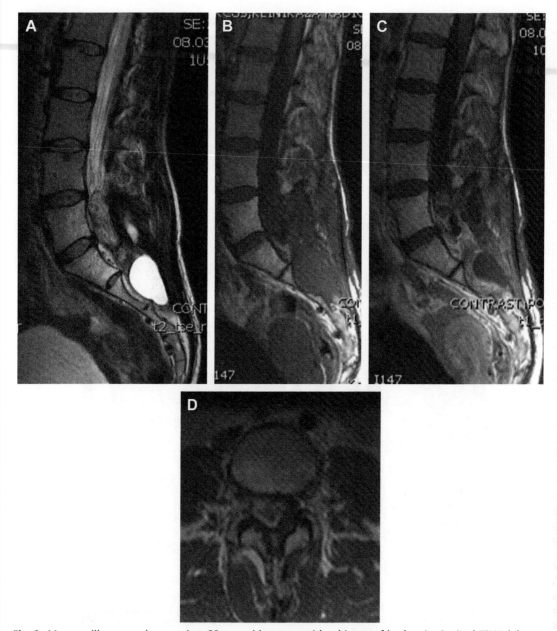

Fig. 2. Myxopapillary ependymoma in a 32-year-old woman with a history of back pain. Sagittal T2WI (*A*), precontrast T1WI (*B*), and contrast-enhanced (*C, D*) T1WI demonstrate a well-defined heterogeneously enhancing cauda equina mass, and an enlarging and remodeling vertebral canal with a large cyst.

HB due to malignant spread of the original primary HB without local recurrence at the surgically resected site.[15]

HB may occur sporadically or in association with von Hippel-Lindau disease.[16]

HBs are low-grade neoplasms, composed of a dense network of vascular capillary channels that contain endothelial cells, pericytes, and lipid-laden stromal cells. Cord HBs are located in the posterior aspect of the spinal cord. They are round, well defined, and usually small. However, they also can be several centimeters in size. "Flow voids" are always present. After contrast administration, small lesions enhance homogeneously, and large lesions heterogeneously. Tumor nodules are usually associated with extensive hydrosyringomyelia (**Fig. 4**). Cysts are often present with variable signal intensity depending on their content. High signal intensity cysts have a high protein content due to previous hemorrhage

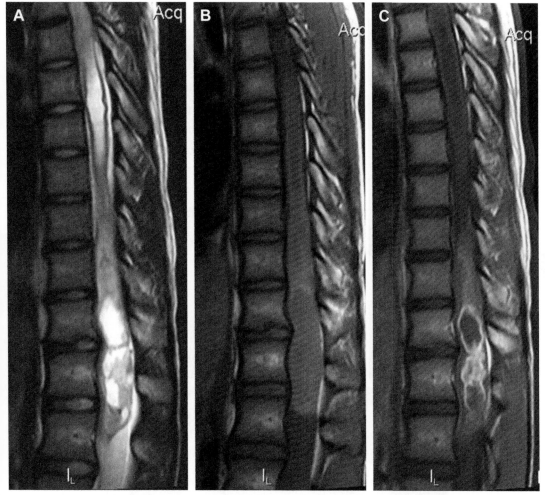

Fig. 3. Pilocytic astrocytoma in a 14-year-old girl with mild low back pain. Sagittal T2-weighted (*A*), STIR (*B*), T1-weighted (*B*), and contrast-enhanced T1-weighted (*C*) MR images of the thoracolumbar spine demonstrate an expanded cord with a large, heterogeneously enhancing tumor with areas of cystic-necrotic degeneration.

or due to transudation of fluid by the tumor itself. When no cystic component is present, extensive edema is usually found. Subarachnoid or even intramedullary hemorrhage caused by spinal cord HB is rare, but should be considered in the differential diagnosis.[17]

Surgery is curative in sporadic cases. The recurrence rate after surgery has been reported to be 15% to 27%, and diffuse spread and disseminated seeding are rarely reported.

Ganglioglioma

Gangliogliomas (WHO grade I) that occur in the spinal cord are extremely rare, and are mostly diagnosed in children and young adults, predominantly localized in the cervical and thoracic spine[18] (**Fig. 5**). Anaplastic gangliogliomas WHO grade III with anaplastic changes in the glial component also have been reported.

Most commonly on MR images, gangliogliomas are seen as circumscribed solid or mixed solid and cystic masses that span a long segment of the cord. Signal intensities are similar to other intramedullary tumors, with low signal on T1WI and high signal on T2WI. Enhancement patterns have been described as highly variable, ranging from minimal to marked, and may be solid, rim, or nodular.[19]

Gangliogliomas WHO grade I are usually cured with gross total resection.

Spinal Cord Metastases

Spinal cord metastases are believed to be rare. More recently, a combination of routine MR imaging and autopsy observation showed that spinal cord metastatic tumors may be more common than initially reported. These rapidly spreading tumors may escape diagnosis, as patients bearing

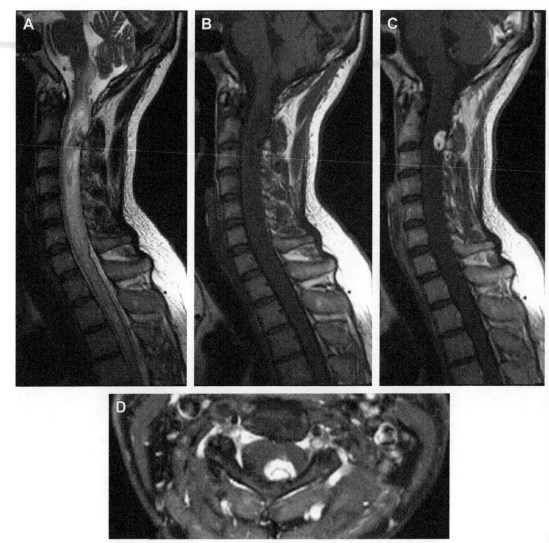

Fig. 4. HB. Sagittal T2WI (*A*), T1WI (*B*), contrast-enhanced sagittal (*C*), and axial (*D*) T1WI demonstrate well-defined, strongly enhancing mass located in the dorsal spinal cord at the C2–C3 level, with associated with edema and extensive syrinx.

these lesions may be asymptomatic. Intramedullary metastases are most common in lung cancer (>50% of cases). Other primary malignancies include breast cancer, melanoma, lymphoma, leukemia, renal cell cancer, and colorectal cancer.

Spinal cord metastases are well-encapsulated masses in the cord, usually eccentrically located with cord expansion. Rarely, they present with cystic changes or intralesional hemorrhage. The most common presentation is a single lesion in the thoracic cord. The mechanism of cord infiltration of a metastatic mass is ambiguous. Because most spinal cord metastases come from the lung, it is thought to be the result of hematogenous dissemination that leads to arterial embolization.

Other proposed theories of tumor seeding involve retrograde infiltration via the spinal cord venous system (Batson plexus), spread through perforating veins in the bone, metastatic antidromic cellular migration via nerve root to the spinal cord, CSF dissemination through intraspinal perineural sheaths, and finally, penetration of the spinal cord parenchyma via penetrating vessels within the Virchow-Robin spaces.[7]

MR imaging is the tool of choice for diagnosing spinal cord metastatic disease. Intramedullary metastases have a nonspecific MR imaging appearance, with cord swelling, edema, and an enhancing lesion. Recently described "rim" and "flame" signs are reportedly useful in the

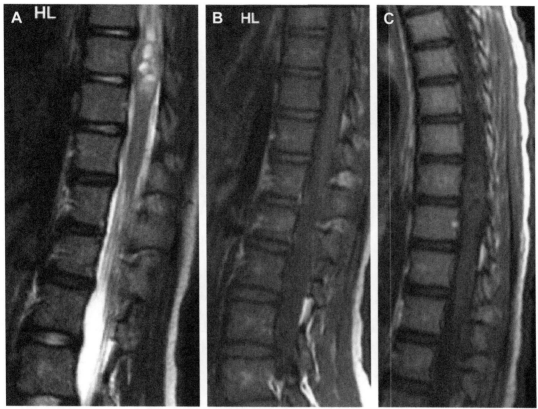

Fig. 5. Ganglioglioma in a 13-year-old girl who presented with a history of mild progressive scoliosis. Sagittal T2WI (*A*), unenhanced (*B*), and contrast-enhanced (*C*) T1WI demonstrate well-defined poorly enhancing mass, with areas of cyst degeneration, at the T8–T10 level.

differentiation of intramedullary metastases and primary spinal cord tumors. The rim sign is defined by Rykken and colleagues[20] as a complete or partial rim of gadolinium enhancement, and the flame sign is defined as an ill-defined, flame-shaped, gadolinium-enhancing region at the superior or inferior margin of an otherwise well-defined lesion.

INTRADURAL-EXTRAMEDULLARY TUMORS
Schwannomas

Schwannomas are the most common benign (WHO grade I) intradural spinal tumors, accounting for 55% of all spinal tumors originating in Schwann cells.[21] Seventy percent of all schwannomas are intradural, whereas 30% can be extradural, and in 15% a dumbbell-shaped (intra I extradural) schwannoma will be found. Schwannomas are more commonly seen in adults, and less commonly in children.

Spinal schwannomas are typically solitary, well-circumscribed, encapsulated masses (**Fig. 6**).[1]

Multiple schwannomas occur in children with neurofibromatosis type 2 (NF-2).[22] NF-2 is an autosomal dominant genetic disorder caused by inactivation of the gene 22q, which acts as a tumor suppressor. Patients with NF-2 develop multiple central and peripheral nervous system tumors, a hallmark unilateral or bilateral vestibular schwannoma, and other cranial and spinal nerve schwannomas, as well as meningiomas and ependymomas.

Schwannomatosis or congenital neurilemmomatosis is a rare syndrome characterized by multiple schwannomas of the peripheral nervous system without involvement of the vestibular nerve. According to the consensus criteria, patients with 2 or more nonintradermal schwannomas, without eighth cranial nerve dysfunction symptoms after the age of 45 years, could be diagnosed as having presumptive schwannomatosis.[23]

On MR imaging, schwannomas are isointense to hypointense on T1WI and isointense to hyperintense on T2WI. Contrast enhancement is moderate to marked and usually homogeneous.

Early surgical resection results in a promising outcome.[24] Only 5% experience local recurrence several years after surgery.[25] According to a

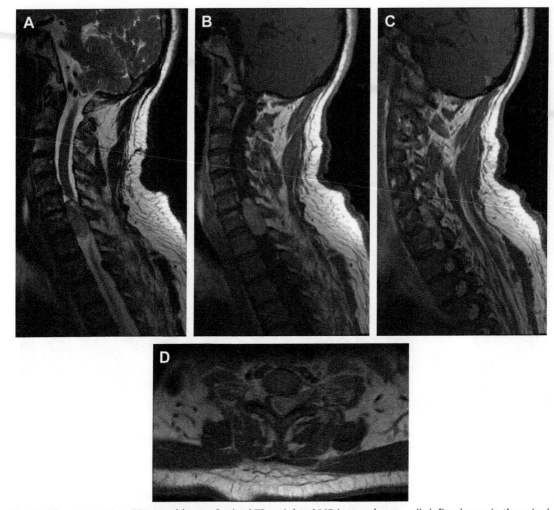

Fig. 6. Schwannoma in a 68-year-old man. Sagittal T2-weighted MR image shows well-defined mass in the spinal canal compressing the cord. (*A*) On sagittal contrast-enhanced T1WIs (*B, C*), intense homogeneous enhancement of a mass is seen. Note the widening of the neural foramen (*C*). Axial postcontrast T1WI (*D*) shows a typical "dumbbell" shape of schwannoma extending intradurally and extradurally.

recently published study, heterogeneously enhancing schwannomas should be followed closely, as they grow more rapidly and may require surgery.[26]

Neurofibromas

Neurofibromas are slow-growing benign tumors (WHO grade I), composed of neoplastic Schwan cells and fibroblasts, without a true capsule. Neurofibromas comprise 5% of all benign soft tissue tumors, and, in 90%, occur as sporadic solitary tumors.[27] Neurofibromas can develop from dorsal spinal nerve roots, as well as peripheral nerves, and in approximately 36% to 40% of patients, in the spinal canal.

Neurofibromas are associated with NF-1. In addition to neurofibromas, *cafe au lait spots,*

axillary freckling, Litsch nodules, optic nerve gliomas, skeletal abnormalities, and malignant peripheral nerve sheath tumors will be present. Patients with neurofibromatosis have an increased risk of developing malignant peripheral nerve sheath tumors, which tend to be more aggressive compared with patients without neurofibromatosis (**Fig. 7**).

Spinal neurofibromas can be identified in 2 different phenotypes of patients with NF-1: (1) classical NF-1 features and only one or a few spinal tumors, and (2) multiple bilateral spinal tumors, but only few NF-1 criteria. The latter has been classified as a subgroup of NF-1, the spinal neurofibromatosis. This may be inherited in an autosomal dominant fashion, called familial spinal neurofibromatosis (FSNF), although this term is also used for sporadic cases.[28]

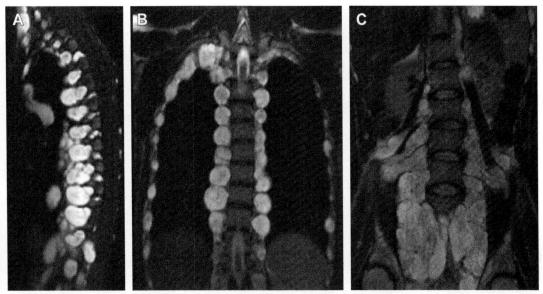

Fig. 7. Multiple neurofibromas in a 29-year-old man with NF-1. Sagittal T2WI (*A*), coronal T2WI (*B*) in the thoracic spine, and coronal T2WI in the lumbar spine (*C*) demonstrate multiple bilateral paraspinal masses.

Neurofibromas are typically recognized as round or fusiform tumors, isointense on T1WI and markedly hyperintense on T2-weighted MR images. On postcontrast images, intense and homogeneous enhancement is seen. However, some neurofibromas will show peripheral enhancement.

At present, the management of spinal neurofibromas consists of careful observation, with resection reserved for the most severe cases. The anatomic location, degree of invasion, and risk of recurrence at the surgical site affect the decision regarding surgery. No definitive chemotherapy has been reported to be successful for plexiform neurofibromas. Rapamycin, imatinib, sorafenib, and interferon have all been used with varying degrees of success.[29]

Meningiomas

Meningiomas are the second most common intraspinal tumor, with the highest incidence in women between 45 and 74 years of age. Asian, Pacific Islander, and Caucasian individuals have the highest frequency of spinal meningiomas.[30] They can occur at any location throughout the spine, but predominate (90% of the cases) in the thoracic region located posterolaterally (**Fig. 8**). Most meningiomas will be intradural and only 10% are extradural or dumbbell tumors. Meningiomas arise from the cells that make up the arachnoid membrane (arachnoid cap cells), and 95% are benign tumors (WHO grade I). Grade II or atypical meningiomas have 4 or more mitotic cells per 10 high-power fields (hpf) and/or 3 or more of the following characteristics: increased

cellularity, small cells, necrosis, prominent nucleoli, sheeting, and/or brain invasion. Grade III (Anaplastic) have 20 or more mitoses per 10 hpf and/or obviously malignant cytologic characteristics. Grade III tumors are often solitary tumors, but, multiple tumors (2%) are associated with NF-2. On imaging, meningiomas are typically round, broad-base masses with a "tail" into the adjacent dura. In 5%, calcifications are present within the tumor, and easily diagnosed on CT. On T1WI and T2WI, they are isointense to the spinal cord and exhibit marked homogeneous enhancement on postcontrast T1WI.

Meningiomas have an excellent prognosis with complete surgical resection in more than 90% of cases.

Hemangiopericytoma

Hemangiopericytomas (HPCs) are rare vascular tumors that arise from pericytes, the contractile cells surrounding capillaries, also known as the pericytes of Zimmermann. This tumor is classified as a grade II tumor. Anaplastic HPC grade III will be diagnosed if the tumor contains infiltrative margins, high cellularity, nuclear pleomorphism, areas of tumor necrosis, and an increased mitotic index. HPCs usually occur in the subcutaneous soft tissue and skeletal system and rarely in the CNS. Meningeal HPCs constitute 2% to 4% of all meningeal tumors and 1% of all CNS tumors.[31] Primary spinal HPCs are divided into intradural and extradural lesions, and intradural are either intramedullary or extramedullary. The extradural lesions are

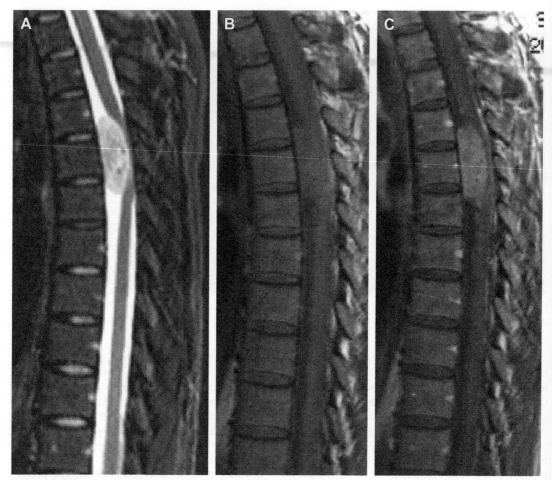

Fig. 8. Meningioma. Sagittal T2-weighted (*A*), T1-weighted (*B*), and contrast-enhanced T1-weighted MR images (*C*) demonstrate a well-circumscribed, homogeneously enhancing intradural-extramedullary lesion in the anterior and left aspect of the spinal canal.

further classified as either dural-based or primarily osseous.[32]

On imaging, HPCs are recognized as multilobular "dumbbell"-shaped masses, expanding and eroding bone. They are hypointense on T1WI, moderately hyperintense on T2WI, with homogeneous enhancement.

HPC has long been considered an aggressive tumor with a poor prognosis. Total resection can be achieved; however, intraoperative bleeding due to the high vascularity of this tumor may be the greatest hindrance. Preoperative embolization is recommended to facilitate surgical resection. Close long-term follow-up is necessary, as local recurrence and distant metastases can develop years after the initial treatment.[33]

Paraganglioma

Paragangliomas (PGs) are neuroendocrine tumors that arise in adrenal and various extra-adrenal locations. Tumors of the carotid body and glomus jugulare constitute more than 90% of reported extra-adrenal PGs. Spinal PGs are rare, slow-growing benign masses (WHO grade I). The age of presentation ranges from 9 to 74 years (mean 46 years), with a slight predominance in male individuals. The vast majority of spinal PGs will be found in the cauda equina region.[34]

On MR imaging, PG is a well-delineated mass, isointense or hypointense compared with the spinal cord on T1WI, hyperintense on T2WI, with a hemosiderin "cap" and marked enhancement. Prominent flow voids and cystic areas can be present. As these imaging characteristics are commonly found in other tumors as well, the diagnosis is rarely made before surgery (**Fig. 9**).

As cauda equina PGs are well-encapsulated tumors, surgical resection is curative in most cases. Radiotherapy is reserved for incompletely resected tumors. Overall, prolonged postoperative

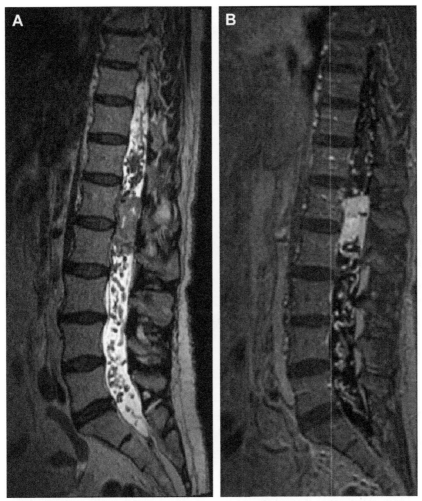

Fig. 9. PG in a 62-year-old woman after tumor embolization. Sagittal T2WI (*A*) and contrast-enhanced T1WI with fat suppression (*B*) demonstrate a well-delineated T2-high signal intensity mass at the L1–2 level. On postcontrast-T1 images (*B*), marked enhancement of the mass and vessels in the spinal canal is observed.

observation is mandatory because of the slow tumor evolution and the possibility of tumor relapse, even up to 30 years after surgery.[35]

Melanocytoma

Meningeal melanocytomas are rare, benign, pigmented tumors of the CNS. Limas and Tio first coined the term "meningeal melanocytoma" in 1972 to describe a pigmented tumor in the foramen magnum region.[36] Most cases of meningeal melanocytomas are found in the intradural-extramedullary compartment, whereas an intramedullary location is rare.[37]

Melanocytomas appear as well-circumscribed or encapsulated pigmented lesions indistinguishable from pigmented meningiomas, schwannomas, and melanomas. Definitive diagnosis is based solely on histopathological and immunohistochemical examination.[36]

Melanocytomas appear as isointense to slightly hyperintense lesions on T1-weighted MRI, isointense to hypointense on T2WI, and demonstrate homogeneous enhancement on postcontrast images.

The optimal treatment for spinal melanocytomas is complete resection.

Melanoma

Primary spinal melanoma is a rare, highly malignant neoplasm, and may be intradural or extradural. The mean age at presentation is 54 years.[38]

On MR imaging, melanoma shows a typical pattern of T1-hyperintensity and T2-hypointensity. These characteristics vary depending on the melanocytic content, and also on intratumoral hemorrhage (**Fig. 10**). Melanoma shows heterogeneous enhancement after contrast administration,

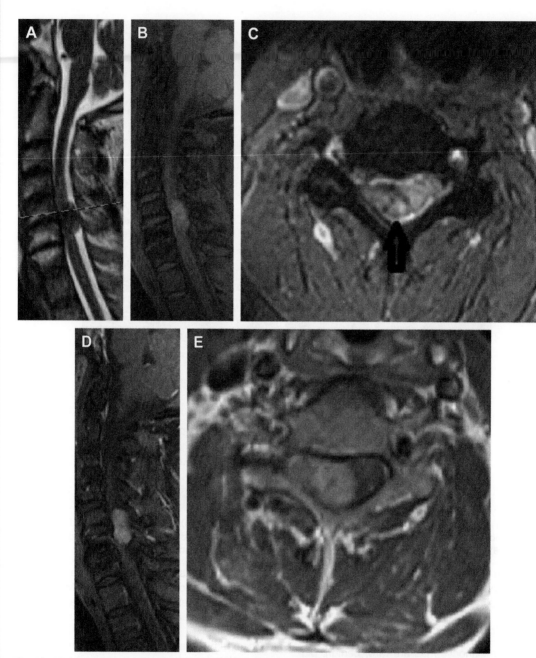

Fig. 10. Melanoma. Sagittal T2WI (*A*), T1WI (*B*), axial T2* (*C*), sagittal (*D*), and axial (*E*) contrast-enhanced T1WI show a T1-high and T2-low signal intensity homogeneously enhancing mass at the C5–C6 level.

with a dural tail sign. Differential diagnosis includes spinal meningioma, meningeal melanocytomas, and metastatic melanoma.

Melanoma is a highly malignant neoplasm, with a median survival rate of 6 to 12 months, and a 5-year survival rate of less than 10%. Complete tumor resection or subtotal resection followed by radiation treatment remains the standard treatment.[39]

Leptomeningeal Metastases

More than 95% of spinal metastases occur in the extradural space, whereas intradural-extramedullary and intramedullary metastases are relatively rare.[40]

Five routes for metastatic intradural spinal tumor spread have been hypothesized: (1) the rich venous plexus, (2) perineural lymphatics, (3) seeding from involved osseous structures to the CSF through the dura, (4) spreading via the subarachnoid space, and (5) hematogenous spreading via the arterial system (Perrin).[41] Drop metastasis is considered to occur as a tertiary metastasis of brain metastasis, induced by the circulation of CSF and gravity in the subarachnoid space.[42]

Leptomeningeal dissemination from CNS neoplasms occurs in younger patients, whereas metastases from lung or breast carcinomas occur in older patients. In children, leptomeningeal spread from medulloblastoma and ependyma is common.[43]

Imaging findings of seeding metastasis include multiple enhanced nodular lesions in the spinal canal and/or a diffuse sheetlike coating of the spinal cord or roots ("carcinomatous meningitis") and thickening of the cauda equina. Unenhanced T1WI and T2WI will be less helpful, as abnormalities are isointense to the spinal cord. Contrast-enhanced T1WIs are mandatory to demonstrate enhancement (**Fig. 11**).

Treatment options for leptomeningeal metastasis are limited. Surgery may be attempted if there is a symptomatic, large metastatic deposit causing cord compression. After the excision of a solitary

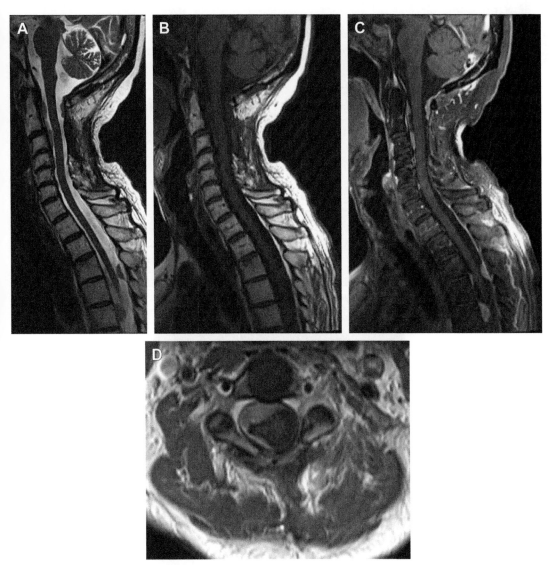

Fig. 11. Leptomeningeal metastases in a 52-year-old man with neuroblastoma. Sagittal T2-weighted (*A*), T1-weighted (*B*), and contrast-enhanced T1-weighted MR images in the sagittal (*C*) and axial (*D*) planes demonstrate multiple nodular enhancing lesions in the spinal canal. Note marked T2-hypointensity (*A*), indicating high cellularity.

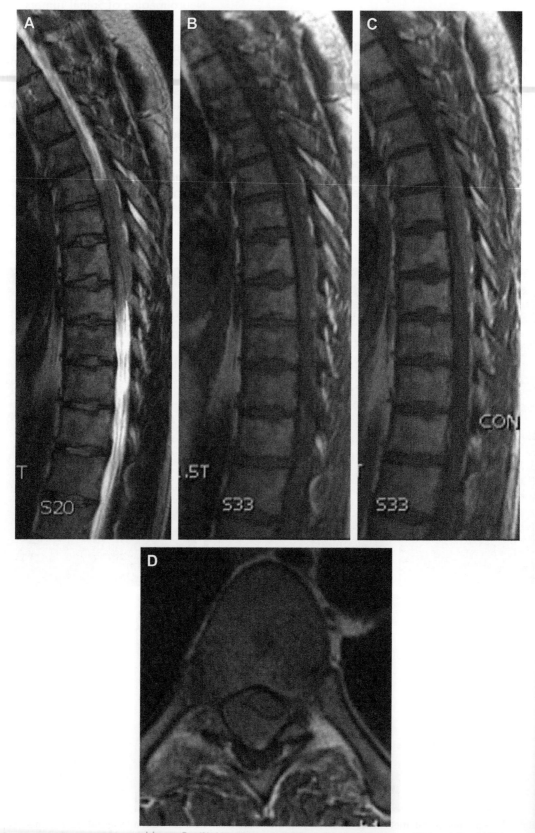

Fig. 12. Lymphoma in 25-year-old man. Sagittal T2WI (*A*), T1WI (*B*), and contrast-enhanced T1-weighted MR images in the sagittal (*C*) and axial (*D*) planes show homogeneously enhancing mass at the T5–8 level in the posterior epidural space, compressing the cord.

metastasis, either a wait-and-scan policy or adjuvant radiation therapy is generally recommended.[44]

LYMPHOMA AND LEUKEMIA
Lymphoma

Most (>85%) of all CNS lymphomas are non-Hodgkin lymphomas, whereas Hodgkin disease is rare. Lymphoma can be located in all of the spinal compartments.

An epidural location for lymphoma is observed in 0.1% to 6.5% of all lymphomas. Epidural lymphoma is a mostly multisegmental mass with isointensity on T1WI, isointense or hyperintense on T2WI, with homogeneous enhancement. Osseous elements may or may not be involved. The most common location for epidural lymphoma is the thoracic spine (Fig. 12).

Lymphomatous involvement of vertebral bodies will be recognized as T1 isointense to slightly hypointense, and T2 isointense to hyperintense lesions with marked high signal on STIR images. Lymphomatous leptomeningitis nearly always occurs as a result of spread from intracranial lymphoma. On MR imaging, thickening of the cauda equina and nerve roots with nodular masses will be present. Primary intramedullary lymphomas of the spine are rare. They can present as a single or as multiple poorly defined enhancing masses.[43]

PET has proved useful for staging and monitoring treatment response in lymphomas. Despite new advances in lymphoma therapies and surgical decompression in cases of epidural lymphoma, the prognosis is still relatively poor. The longest survival period has been reported for primary osseous lymphoma (10-year survival rate approximately 90%).[45]

Leukemia

Both acute and chronic myeloid or lymphoid leukemia may present with spinal involvement. Single or multiple vertebral bodies can be affected with diffuse osteopenia, multiple compression fractures, and meningeal infiltration.

Leukemic meningitis is usually seen in acute lymphatic leukemia, and occurs without systemic disease in 18%, and during remission in 36%. Patients present with lower extremity weakness, numbness, and pain. Lumbar puncture with CSF analysis is necessary to exclude other pathologies. On MR imaging, pial enhancement of the spinal cord ("sugar coating") will be seen.

Myeloid sarcoma (chloroma) is a rare, extramedullary tumor of immature myeloid cells, with a less than 1% frequency in the spine. It could occur concomitantly, or, rarely, before the onset of systemic bone marrow involvement.[46] Sarcomas can be the initial manifestation of leukemia or occur during a remission or relapse period. The lumbosacral and thoracic portions of the spine are reported to be commonly involved.[47] This highly vascularized mass is composed of immature granulocytes, and is, therefore, also called granulocytic sarcoma. On MR imaging, they are isointense to hyperintense on T1WI, isointense to hypointense on T2WI, and show moderate to marked gadolinium enhancement.

On MRI, leukemic marrow has a high signal on T1WI and T2WI, with abnormal enhancement on postcontrast images.

Rarely, leukemia my present as an epidural mass, and it must be considered in the differential diagnosis of a spinal epidural mass.[48]

Chemotherapy, radiation therapy, and bone marrow transplantation are treatment options.

REFERENCES

1. Duong LM, McCarthy BJ, McLendon RE, et al. Descriptive epidemiology of malignant and nonmalignant primary spinal cord, spinal meninges, and cauda equina tumors, United States, 2004–2007. Cancer 2012;118(17):4220–7.
2. Landi A, Palmarini V, D'Elia A, et al. Magnetic resonance diffusion tensor imaging and fiber-tracking diffusion tensor tractography in the management of spinal astrocytomas. World J Clin Cases 2016;4(1):1–4.
3. Alkherayf F, Arab AF, Tsai E. Conus medullaris teratoma with utilization of fiber tractography: case report. J Neurol Surg Rep 2015;76(1):183–7.
4. Krings T, Lasjaunias PL, Hans FJ, et al. Imaging in spinal vascular disease. Neuroimaging Clin N Am 2007;17:57–72.
5. Naito K, Yamagata T, Arima H, et al. Qualitative analysis of spinal intramedullary lesions using PET/CT. J Neurosurg Spine 2015;31:1–7.
6. Louis DN, Ohgaki H, Wiestler OD, et al. The 2007 WHO classification of tumours of the central nervous system. Acta Neuropathol 2007;114(2):97–109.
7. Samartzis D, Gillis CC, Shih P, et al. Intramedullary spinal cord tumors: part I-epidemiology, pathophysiology, and diagnosis. Global Spine J 2015;5(5):425–35.
8. Chen X, Li C, Che X, et al. Spinal myxopapillary ependymomas: a retrospective clinical and immunohistochemical study. Acta Neurochir (Wien) 2016;158(1):101–7.
9. Tomek M, Jayajothi A, Brandner S, et al. Imaging features of spinal tanycytic ependymoma. Neuroradiol J 2016;29(1):61–5.
10. Oh MC, Tarapore PE, Kim JM, et al. Spinal ependymomas: benefits of extent of resection for different

histological grades. J Clin Neurosci 2013;20(10): 1390–7.

11. Huisman TA. Pediatric tumors of the spine. Cancer Imaging 2009;2(9):45–8.

12. Ruppert B, Welsh CT, Hannah J, et al. Glioneuronal tumor with neuropil-like islands of the spinal cord with diffuse leptomeningeal neuraxis dissemination. J Neurooncol 2011;104(2):529–33.

13. Marko NF, Weil RJ. The molecular biology of WHO grade I astrocytomas. Neuro Oncol 2012;14(12): 1424–31.

14. Yagi T, Ohata K, Haque M, et al. Intramedullary spinal cord tumour associated with neurofibromatosis type 1. Acta Neurochir (Wien) 1997;139(11): 1055–60.

15. Choyke PL, Glenn GM, Walther MM, et al. von Hippel-Lindau disease: genetic, clinical, and imaging features. Radiology 1995;194:629–42.

16. Chung SY, Jeun SS, Park JH. Disseminated hemangioblastoma of the central nervous system without Von Hippel-Lindau disease. Brain Tumor Res Treat 2014;2(2):96–101.

17. Koda M, Mannoji C, Itabashi T, et al. Intramedullary hemorrhage caused by spinal cord hemangioblastoma: a case report. BMC Res Notes 2014;7:823.

18. Gessi M, Dörner E, Dreschmann V, et al. Intramedullary gangliogliomas: histopathologic and molecular features of 25 cases. Hum Pathol 2016;49:107–13.

19. Oppenheimer DC, Johnson MD, Judkins AR. Ganglioglioma of the spinal cord. J Clin Imaging Sci 2015;5:53.

20. Rykken JB, Diehn FE, Hunt CH, et al. Rim and flame signs: postgadolinium MRI findings specific for non-CNS intramedullary spinal cord metastases. AJNR Am J Neuroradiol 2013;34(4):908–15.

21. Hirano K, Imagama S, Sato K, et al. Primary spinal cord tumors: review of 678 surgically treated patients in Japan. A multicenter study. Eur Spine J 2012;21:2019–26.

22. Evans DG. Neurofibromatosis type 2 (NF2): A clinical and molecular review. Orphanet J Rare Dis 2009;4:16.

23. MacCollin M, Chiocca EA, Evans DG, et al. Diagnostic criteria for schwannomatosis. Neurology 2005;64:1838–45.

24. Deng Q, Tian Z, Sheng W, et al. Surgical methods and efficacies for cervicothoracolumbar spinal schwannoma. Exp Ther Med 2015;10(6):2023–8.

25. Fehlings MG, Nater A, Zamorano JJ, et al. Risk factors for recurrence of surgically treated conventional spinal schwannomas: analysis of 169 patients from a multicenter international database. Spine (Phila Pa 1976) 2016;41(5):390–8.

26. Ando K, Imagama S, Ito Z, et al. How do spinal schwannomas progress? The natural progression of spinal schwannomas on MRI. J Neurosurg Spine 2016;24(1):155–9.

27. Chen MZ. Neurofibroma. In: Ross JS, et al, editors. Diagnostic imaging. Spine. 1st edition. Salt Lake City (UT): Amirsys; 2004. p. IV-1-90. IV-1-93.

28. Upadhyaya M, Spurlock G, Kluwe L, et al. The spectrum of somatic and germline NF1 mutations in NF1 patients with spinal neurofibromas. Neurogenetics 2009;10:251–63.

29. Carman KB, Yakut A, Anlar B, et al. Spinal neurofibromatosis associated with classical neurofibromatosis type 1: genetic characterization of an atypical case. BMJ Case Rep 2013;14:2013.

30. Kshettry VR, Hsieh JK, Ostrom QT, et al. Descriptive epidemiology of spinal meningiomas in the United States. Spine (Phila Pa 1976) 2015;40(15): 886–9.

31. Liu HG, Yang AC, Chen N, et al. Hemangiopericytomas in the spine: clinical features, classification, treatment, and long-term follow-up in 26 patients. Neurosurgery 2013;72:16–24.

32. Ramdasi RV, Nadkarni TD, Goel NA. Hemangiopericytoma of the cervical spine. J Craniovertebr Junction Spine 2014;5(2):95–8.

33. Zhang P, Hu J, Zhou D. Hemangiopericytoma of the cervicothoracic spine: a case report and literature review. Turk Neurosurg 2014;24(6): 948–53.

34. Mishra T, Goel NA, Goel AH. Primary paraganglioma of the spine: A clinicopathological study of eight cases. J Craniovertebr Junction Spine 2014;5(1): 20–4.

35. Corinaldesi R, Novegno F, Giovenali P, et al. Paraganglioma of the cauda equina region. Spine J 2015;15(3):e1–8.

36. Dorwal P, Mohapatra I, Gautam D, et al. Intramedullary melanocytoma of thoracic spine: a rare case report. Asian J Neurosurg 2014;9(1):36–9.

37. Karikari IO, Powers CJ, Bagley CA, et al. Primary intramedullary melanocytoma of the spinal cord: case report. Neurosurgery 2009;64(4):E777–8.

38. Trinh V, Medina-Flores R, Taylor CL, et al. Primary melanocytic tumors of the central nervous system: report of two cases and review of literature. Surg Neurol Int 2014;5:147.

39. Li YP, Zhang HZ, She L, et al. Primary extramedullary spinal melanoma mimicking spinal meningioma: a case report and literature review. Oncol Lett 2014; 8(1):339–44.

40. Takeuchi K, Hagiwara Y, Kanaya K, et al. Drop metastasis of adrenocorticotropic hormone-producing pituitary carcinoma to the cauda equina. Asian Spine J 2014;8(5):680–3.

41. Perrin RG, Livingston KE, Aarabi B. Intradural extramedullary spinal metastasis. A report of 10 cases. J Neurosurg 1982;56:835–7.

42. Lee CH, Kim KJ, Hyun SJ, et al. Intradural extramedullary metastasis of small cell lung cancer: a case report. Korean J Spine 2012;9(3):293–6.

43. Abul-Kasim K, Thurnher MM, McKeever P, et al. Intradural spinal tumors: current classification and MRI features. Neuroradiology 2008;50(4):301–14.

44. Shah A, Redhu R, Nadkarni T, et al. Supratentorial glioblastoma multiforme with spinal metastases. J Craniovertebr Junction Spine 2010;1:126–9.

45. Katzman GL. Lymphoma. In: Ross JS, et al, editors. Diagnostic imaging spine. 1st edition. Salt Lake City (UT): Amirsys; 2004. p. IV-1-54. IV-1-57.

46. Hu X, Shahab I, Lieberman IH. Spinal myeloid sarcoma "chloroma" presenting as cervical radiculopathy: case report. Global Spine J 2015;5(3):241–6.

47. Seok JH, Park J, Kim SK, et al. Granulocytic sarcoma of the spine: MRI and clinical review. AJR Am J Roentgenol 2010;194(2):485–9.

48. Higashida T, Kawasaki T, Sakata K, et al. Acute lymphocytic leukemia recurring in the spinal epidural space. Neurol Med Chir (Tokyo) 2007;47(8):375–8.

Imaging in Spondylodiskitis

Elena Prodi, MD[a], Roberto Grassi, MD[b], Francesca Iacobellis, MD[b],
Alessandro Cianfoni, MD[a],*

KEYWORDS

- Spondylodiskitis • Imaging • Infection • Biopsy • Spine

KEY POINTS

- MR imaging is the imaging modality of choice for the diagnosis of spondylodiskitis, from early diagnosis to follow-up.
- Typical findings of spondylodiskitis are abnormal low signal on T1-weighted images and high signal on fat-suppressed T2-weighted images of the disk and opposing vertebral bodies, with contrast enhancement, associated with erosion and destruction of the vertebral end plates.
- Soft tissue involvement is a key finding that helps differentiate spondylodiskitis from other common conditions, such as Modic type I degenerative end plate changes and erosive intervertebral osteochondrosis.
- An image-guided biopsy is recommended in all patients with suspected spondylodiskitis based on clinical, laboratory, and imaging studies, when a microbiologic diagnosis has not been established by blood cultures.

DISCUSSION OF PROBLEM/CLINICAL PRESENTATION

Infectious spondylitis represents 2% to 7% of cases of skeletal infection. Spondylodikcitis (SD) shows a bimodal age distribution, with a peak below 20 years and another peak between 50 and 70 years. A 2:1 to 5:1 male/female ratio has been reported.[1] Risk factors include a remote infection (present in about 25% of cases), spinal interventions, trauma, intravenous drug abuse, advanced age, diabetes mellitus, immunosuppression (long-term systemic administration of steroids, organ transplantation, human immunodeficiency virus), malnutrition, and cancer.[2] The incidence of SD has increased in recent years as a consequence of improved life expectancy, comorbid factors, and higher number of spinal interventions. Postsurgical diskitis represents up to 30% of all cases of pyogenic SD.[3]

SD can occur anywhere in the vertebral column but the most common site is the lumbar spine (58%), followed by the thoracic spine (30%), and the cervical spine (11%), with single level involvement (65%), multiple contiguous levels (20%), and multiple noncontiguous levels (10%).[4]

Since the advent of antibiotics, mortality has dropped to less than 5%.[5] The morbidity of SD is significant and is related to spinal deformity with chronic pain and possible neurologic deficits.

The causative agents are mainly bacteria, less commonly fungi and parasites. The most common cause of pyogenic SD is hematogenous spread of *Staphylococcus aureus* (60%), followed by *Enterobacter* species (30%). Other pyogenic agents may be encountered, such as *Salmonella*, *Klebsiella*, *Pseudomonas*, and *Streptococcus*.[6] Nonpyogenic infections originate from *Mycobacterium tuberculosis*, *Brucella*, fungi, and parasites. Human

The authors have nothing to disclose.
[a] Department of Neuroradiology, Neurocenter of Southern Switzerland, Via Tesserete 46, Lugano 6900, Switzerland; [b] Department of Radiology, Second University of Naples, Piazza Miraglia 2, Naples 80138, Italy
* Corresponding author.
E-mail address: alessandro.cianfoni@eoc.ch

Magn Reson Imaging Clin N Am 24 (2016) 581–600
http://dx.doi.org/10.1016/j.mric.2016.04.005
1064-9689/16/$ – see front matter © 2016 Elsevier Inc. All rights reserved.

mri.theclinics.com

immunodeficiency virus infections have caused an increase in incidence of SD from *M tuberculosis* (Pott disease) in recent years. Fungal infections (*Cryptococcus neoformans*, *Candida* species, *Histoplasma capsulatum*, *Coccidioides immitis*) are rare and associated with immunodepression.[7]

Persistent back or neck pain, malaise, fever, anorexia, tenderness, and rigidity may be the presenting symptom. A more insidious onset with nonspecific pain and malaise is also possible. The presence of fever is inconstant, reported in 35% to 60%[4,8] possibly related to common intake of analgesic drugs. Signs of nerve root compression with radiculopathy, meningeal irritation, lower extremity weakness, or paraplegia can be present with epidural involvement. Difficulty in swallowing and torticollis may be present in patients with cervical location. The onset of symptoms may be indolent and there is often a delay of 2 to 12 weeks in diagnosis.[9] In children clinical presentation is even less specific, including failure or refusal to walk, abdominal pain, chronic back pain, irritability, incontinence, and local tenderness. Fever is rare.[10]

Laboratory findings include elevation of erythrocyte sedimentation rate and C-reactive protein (CRP) that are sensitive, although nonspecific, infection markers. CRP normalization is a useful marker to monitor treatment response.[11] The white blood cell count has low sensitivity.[12]

PATHOLOGY AND RELEVANT ANATOMY
Hematogenous Arterial Spread

Hematogenous arterial spread is the most recognized route of infection. The disk space is rather avascular in adults, whereas it is penetrated by anastomotic vessels in children.[13] End plates provide nutrients to the disk of adults through simple diffusion. The disk end plates are highly vascular, whereas posterior vertebral elements have lower vascularity. The richest arteriolar network is located in the subchondral regions of the vertebral body, which is the equivalent of the metaphysis of a long bone. Hematogenous spread occurs at the end arterioles adjacent to the end plates posterior to the anterior longitudinal ligament. Septic emboli induce bone infarcts and infection in the end plate, whereas the disk space is usually secondarily involved by the enzymatic damage activity of pathogens. However, because of lack of immediate blood defense mechanisms in the disk, infection rapidly establishes. Spreading to the posterior vertebral structures is rare because of their minor vascular supply, and occurs more frequently in fungal and tubercular SD. In children, because of vascularity of disk spaces, the infection may be

located first within the disk. In tubercular SD there is typical involvement of the anterior part of the inferior end plate, spread beneath the anterior longitudinal ligament to the superior end plate of the adjacent vertebra, and possible formation of subligamentous and intraosseous abscess. The disk is spared until late phases.[14] Hematogenous venous spread throughout the venous plexus of Batson is also a possible but less recognized route of infection.[15]

Contiguous Tissues Spread

A contiguous tissue spread is rare and may occur in the context of adjacent infection, including esophageal ruptures, retropharyngeal abscesses, or infections of aortic implants.[16]

Direct Inoculation

Direct inoculation is frequently iatrogenic: postsurgical, more rarely after lumbar puncture, epidural, or intradiskal injections.[3] Other sources are penetrating trauma, direct exposure related to skin breakdown, or open wounds.

IMAGING MODALITIES AND PROTOCOLS
Radiography

Plain radiographs have low sensitivity and specificity, especially in the early phases.[17]

Computed Tomography

Nonenhanced computed tomography (CT) provides excellent evaluation of bone changes, detects gas and calcifications, and contrast-enhanced CT allows evaluation of associated paraspinal and to a lesser extent of epidural soft tissue involvement. CT is inaccurate in evaluating disk spaces, intradural compartment, and neural elements. CT is also routinely used for guidance in percutaneous needle biopsy.

MR Imaging

MR imaging is the imaging of choice in all phases of the disease because of high sensitivity, specificity, and accuracy (96%, 92%, and 94%, respectively).[18] With multiplanar T1-weighted, fat-suppressed T2-weighted, and fat-suppressed contrast-enhanced T1-weighted sequences, as routinely performed, on high field (1.5–3.0 T) magnets, MR imaging offers excellent depiction of bone edema, disk inflammation, paraspinal and epidural soft tissue involvement, compression of neural structures, and intradural compartment spread. It is important that T2-weighted and enhanced T1-weighted images are acquired with fat-suppression, otherwise even extensive inflammatory lesions might result as invisible.[19] Diffusion-weighted spinal imaging (DWI) might help differentiate acute SD from degenerative Modic type I changes[20,21] but its clinical use is still debated.

Nuclear Medicine

Three-phase technetium-99m scintigraphy is sensitive (90%) but nonspecific (78%) in SD. Specificity may be increased by combining technetium-99m scintigraphy with gallium-67[22] or performing a scan with indium-111 labeled white blood cells that accumulate in areas of inflammation. The spatial resolution is low and the detection of epidural abscess is inferior compared with MR imaging. These techniques are therefore reserved for patients with contraindication to MR imaging or when MR imaging is inconclusive. PET scanning with 18 F-fluorodeoxyglucose has a diagnostic accuracy similar to that of MR imaging. However, this technique is not widely available[23] and offers less anatomic information; PET-CT can be used as a problem-solving technique in selected cases.

IMAGING FINDINGS
Imaging in the Acute Phase (<3 Weeks)

Radiography

Radiographs are typically negative for 2 to 3 weeks after the onset of infection (**Fig. 1**). The earliest

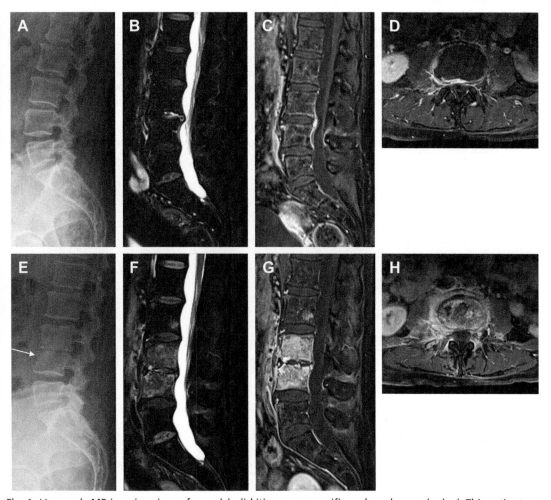

Fig. 1. Very early MR imaging signs of spondylodiskitis are nonspecific and can be overlooked. This patient presented with low back pain for 3 weeks and mildly elevated inflammatory markers. The first plain films (*A*) were unremarkable; MR imaging (*B, D*) showed high T2 signal (*B*) and focal contrast enhancement (*C, D*) in the anulus fibrosis and end plate at L3-L4. Untreated, the back pain worsened; follow-up plain films 3 weeks later (*E*) showed disk space narrowing and loss of definition of the end plates' cortex (*arrow*). MR imaging (*F–H*) showed typical findings of spondylodiskitis, with edema and enhancement of the opposed vertebral bodies and of the adjacent perivertebral soft tissue, also visible on axial fat-suppressed enhanced T1-weighted image (*H*).

radiographic sign is loss of definition, irregularity, and hazy porotic changes of the vertebral end plate related to depletion of the bony matrix, usually starting anterosuperiorly.

Computed tomography

CT scans may appear normal in the early phases of disease. Subtle areas of erosion or osseous destruction may be visible.

MR imaging

MR imaging is the most sensitive imaging method, showing osseous edema, caused by inflammation, as low signal on T1-weighted and high signal on fat-suppressed T2-weighted images, with common contrast-enhancement of the disk and adjacent vertebral bodies visible on fat-suppressed postcontrast T1-weighted images (see **Fig. 1**). The disk, after an initial and rarely seen increase of height, shows height reduction and typically shows loss or distortion of the internuclear cleft, a normal anatomic structure that seems to be a constant feature in subjects 30 years of age or older.[24] In children, infection usually involves the disk primarily and the infected disk shows decreased T2-signal intensity.

Imaging in the Subacute Phase (3 Weeks– 3 Months)

Radiography

Typical signs are progressive erosive osteolysis and osteopenia of end plates, and disk space narrowing (see **Fig. 1**). The presence of a paraspinal mass is visible as thickened retropharyngeal space in cervical SD, displacement of the parietal pleura in thoracic SD, and indistinct margins of the psoas muscle in lumbar SD.

Computed tomography

Typical findings are loss of disk height with disk hypodensity, erosion of end plates cortex, subperiosteal defects, and osteopenia (**Fig. 2**). Marked osseous erosion and destruction of the end plates might actually give the appearance of a widened intervertebral space (**Fig. 3**). The vertebral body erosions are caused by inflammation and by necrosis from obstruction of the vascular supply to the bone. Soft tissue involvement might be

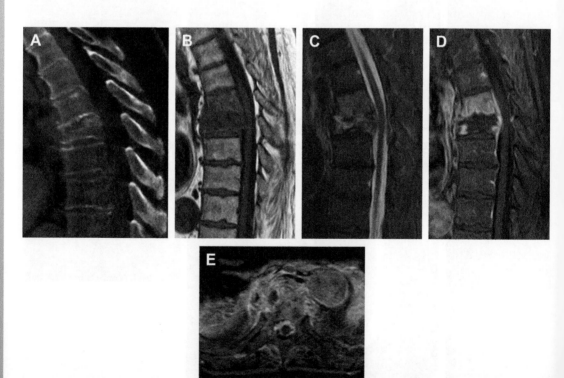

Fig. 2. A patient with history of intravenous drug abuse presented with 6 weeks history of thoracic back rigidity and tenderness. Unenhanced CT (*A*) showed wedge deformity of a midthoracic vertebral body, with adjacent disk space narrowing and cortical irregularity and fraying of the superior end plate. MR imaging showed edema on T1-weighted (*B*) and short tau inversion recovery (STIR) (*C*) images, with contrast enhancement of adjacent vertebral bodies and perivertebral soft tissue on fat-suppressed enhanced T1-weighted images (*D*, *E*). There is thickening and enhancement, with no fluid necrotic components, in the ventral epidural space, likely combination of early phlegmon and epidural venous congestion, concurring to initial spinal cord compression.

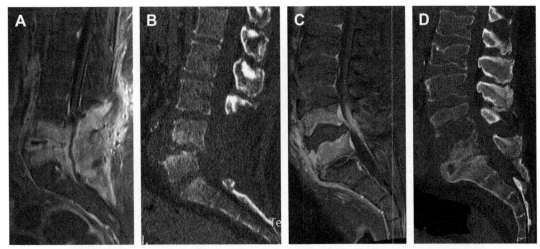

Fig. 3. In the subacute phase CT exquisitely shows osseous changes of spondylodiskitis. In the first case (*A, B*) there were mixed phenomena of cortical irregularities, bony resorption, and subchondral sclerosis along the L4-L5 end plates. In the second case (*C, D*) the CT showed to much better extent the degree of osseous destruction of the cortical and spongious subchondral bone on the opposed sides of the L4-L5 disk space.

visible as obliteration of fat planes and swelling. Gas component may be visible within the disk, the vertebral body, and the paraspinal soft tissues, but has low specificity because it is commonly observed also in degenerative noninfectious conditions (**Fig. 4**). Epidural extension of the disease can be depicted. Soft tissue calcification may be visible in tubercular SD.

MR imaging

The typical findings in SD are high T2 signal and contrast enhancement of the disk and adjacent bone marrow, with almost invariable involvement of paraspinal and epidural soft tissues (see **Figs. 1–3**). The infection extending to the epidural space and to the paraspinal soft tissues causes phlegmon or abscesses (see later). Infection may cause engorgement of epidural basivertebral veins by direct extension of the inflammatory process, by mechanical obstruction to venous drainage, or by both (see **Fig. 2**). However, prominence and contrast enhancement of the epidural venous plexus should not be confused with epidural infection. Disk height loss is visible when present.

Imaging in the Chronic Phase (>3 Months) and Sequelae of Spondylodiskitis

Radiography

After approximately 10 weeks, plain radiographs may show reactive sclerosis, new bone formation with osteophytosis, kyphotic deformity, scoliosis, spondylolisthesis, and bony ankylosis.

Computed tomography

Osseous changes described previously related to SD are better depicted with CT (**Fig. 5**).

MR imaging

Signs of edema and contrast enhancement gradually resolve, leaving behind sclerotic changes, with low T1 and T2 signal, sometimes with minimal residual contrast enhancement. Vertebral body height changes, kyphosis, scoliosis, spondylolisthesis, and ankylosis can all be seen during the late/healing stage of the infectious process (see **Fig. 5**). In infants, SD may present as progressive dissolution of involved vertebral bodies without loss of disk height. Years later, the kyphotic deformity from this infection may mimic congenital kyphosis.

Epidural Spread

Infections in the epidural space is a threatening condition because of the risk of spinal cord injury, either from direct compression, or because of thrombosis or thrombophlebitis of epidural veins and consequent spinal cord infarction. Severe back pain associated with progressive neurologic deficit and fever are the most common symptoms. Laboratory studies show elevated erythrocyte sedimentation rate and CRP; leukocytosis may be present. MR imaging is the modality of choice to investigate epidural infections. A phlegmon must be distinguished from an abscess. Phlegmons appear as ill-defined soft tissues changes, hypointense on T1-weighted and hyperintense on T2-weighted images, in the

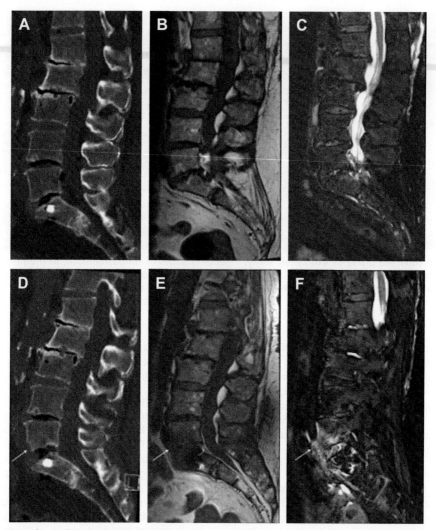

Fig. 4. A patient who underwent surgical hardware fixation of a sacral and pelvic fracture had a postoperative CT (*A*) and MR imaging (*B, C*) showing multilevel degenerative disk pathology with disk space narrowing and gas vacuum. Four weeks later because of worsening low back pain a follow-up CT was obtained, showing interval erosion of the anteroinferior corner of the L5 vertebral body (*arrow on D*); subsequent MR imaging showed to much better extent the edematous changes across L5-S1 disk space (*arrows on E and F*), on T1-weighted (*E*) and STIR (*F*) images, strongly suggesting spondylodiskitis. As in this case, presence of gas can be seen in spondylodiskitis, but has no specificity.

perivertebral and epidural spaces, with little mass effect, and homogeneous contrast enhancement (**Fig. 6**). Abscesses are characterized by a necrotic center, hyperintense on T2-weighted images, isointense to hypointense on T1-weighted images, with linear thin or thick enhancing peripheral rim, and usually exert mass effect if in the epidural space. DWI can show restricted diffusion (visible as brilliant hyperintense signal on b500–800, and low signal on ADC maps) in the pyogenic abscess cavity.[25] A phlegmon reflects hyperhemia and inflammation, is not drainable, and can be treated pharmacologically,

whereas an abscess might require urgent percutaneous or surgical drainage, especially when in the epidural space (**Fig. 7**).

Paraspinal Abscesses

Contiguous spread of infection from the spine to the adjacent soft tissues may result in the formation of abscesses in the paraspinal and psoas muscles, retroperitoneum, and subpleuric space that appear as unilobulated or multilobulated fluid-filled expansile lesions, hypointense on T1-weighted and hyperintense on T2-weighted

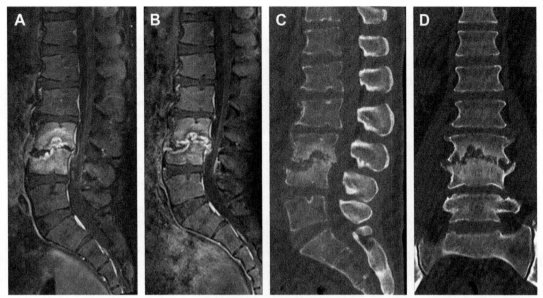

Fig. 5. In the late healing phase, MR imaging findings slowly regress, but some degree of edema and enhancement along end plates and opposed vertebral bodies (*A*, *B*) can persist beyond clinical resolution and normalization of inflammatory markers. CT shows the final result of the stabilized osseous abnormalities, such as destruction, sclerosis, osteophytes, ankylosis, deformity, and pseudoarthrosis (*C*, *D*).

images, with rim enhancement after contrast administration (**Fig. 8**). The incidence of abscess formation is higher in granulomatous infections. The presence of such an abscess may require CT-guided drainage.

Facet Joint Infection

Facet joint septic arthritis is a rare form of spinal infection that has to be considered in patients with febrile spinal syndromes. The route of infection to the facet joint is more commonly

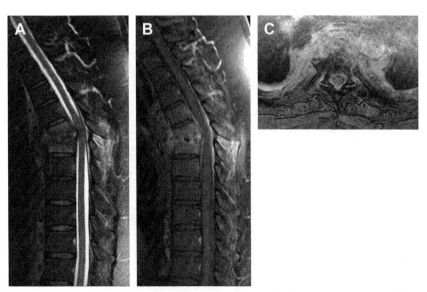

Fig. 6. The difference between a phlegmon and an abscess is crucial because they have different treatment options. In this case of midthoracic spondylodiskitis the combination of vertebral destruction leading to deformity and focal kyphosis, and the circumferential thickening of the epidural soft tissues caused spinal cord compression (*A*). On fat-suppressed contrast-enhanced T1-weighted images (*B*, *C*) the enhancement in the epidural space is homogeneous, with no evidence of drainable fluid-filled cavities, referable to as epidural phlegmon rather than abscess. Surgical decompression, debridement, and stabilization was urgently performed.

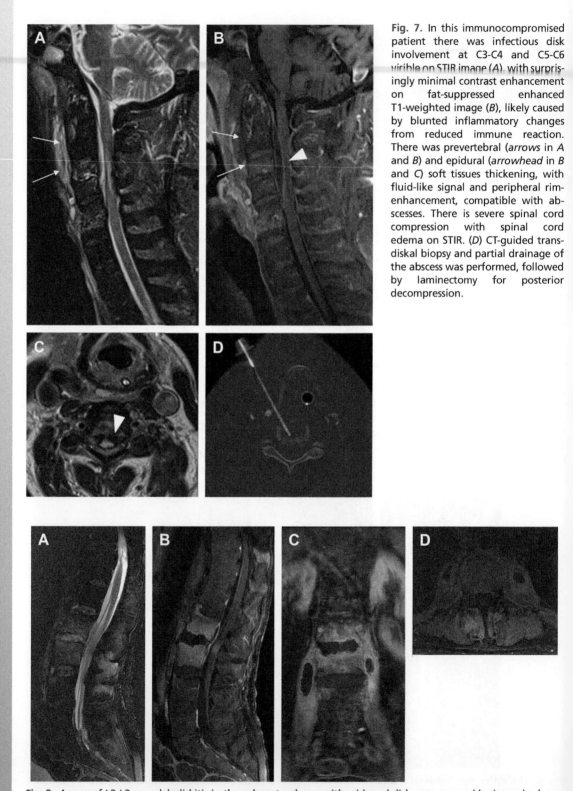

Fig. 7. In this immunocompromised patient there was infectious disk involvement at C3-C4 and C5-C6 visible on STIR image (A), with surprisingly minimal contrast enhancement on fat-suppressed enhanced T1-weighted image (B), likely caused by blunted inflammatory changes from reduced immune reaction. There was prevertebral (arrows in A and B) and epidural (arrowhead in B and C) soft tissues thickening, with fluid-like signal and peripheral rim-enhancement, compatible with abscesses. There is severe spinal cord compression with spinal cord edema on STIR. (D) CT-guided transdiskal biopsy and partial drainage of the abscess was performed, followed by laminectomy for posterior decompression.

Fig. 8. A case of L2-L3 spondylodiskitis in the subacute phase, with widened disk space caused by irregular bony resorption of the end plates, diffuse contrast enhancement of the opposed vertebral bodies, and early involvement of the disk level above (A, B). Extensive contrast enhancement was visible in the psoas and paraspinal muscles (C, D). Abscess cavities were also present in both psoas muscles, amenable to CT-guided drainage. A small epidural abscess is also visible behind L2-L3 bodies (A, B).

nonhematogenous because the vascular supply of the facet joints differs from that of vertebral body. Involvement is unilateral or bilateral through possible diffusion via the retrodural space of Okada. MR imaging represents the imaging modality of choice showing high T2 signal of the pus fluid–filled joint capsule, with peripheral enhancement, and soft tissue and adjacent osseous edema (**Fig. 9**). CT demonstrates erosive changes, loss of density of ligamentum flavum, and obliteration of fat planes.[26] This constellation of findings overlaps with acute noninfectious inflammatory changes of degenerative conditions. Posterior epiduritis, pyomyositis, or the presence of an abscess in the paraspinal muscles or psoas muscle can be associated.

Pearls, Pitfalls, and Variants: Typical Imaging Pattern in Pyogenic, Tubercular, Brucella, and Fungal Spondylodiskitis

Some imaging features can strongly support the differential diagnosis of spinal infection etiologies.

Pyogenic[27]
- The favorite location is the lumbar spine, with adjacent vertebral levels involved.
- Vertebral body involvement is present and normally starts from the anterior portion.
- Disk involvement is present in the early stage.
- Paraspinal/epidural space involvement may be present, with inflammation and/or small abscesses with thick and irregular rim enhancement.
- Posterior elements are typically not involved.
- Anterior subligamentous spread is uncommon.

Tubercular[28–30]
- Tubercular SD typically shows an indolent clinical course with gradual onset of symptoms over months to a year.
- The favorite location is the thoracic/thoracolumbar junction, with adjacent vertebral and multilevel involvement and presence of skip lesions in 4% of cases.
- Vertebral body involvement is characterized by prominent destruction of the anterior aspect of the vertebral body, disk space sparing until late in the course of the disease, with wedging, often leading to gibbus deformity. Posterior elements may be involved with higher frequency compared with pyogenic SD. Infection limited to a single vertebral body may cause vertebral collapse and vertebra plana. Ivory vertebra may result from reossification of the bone as a healing response to osteonecrosis. Typical findings of tuberculous spondylitis include bony fragmentation, intersegmental fusions, and intraosseous vertebral abscess with ring enhancement (**Fig. 10**).
- Disk involvement is variable, from sparing to severe destruction; this may be caused by a relative lack of proteolytic enzymes in tuberculosis, but when both vertebral end plates are involved, the disk may lose its source of nutrition and become involved secondarily.
- Paraspinal/epidural space involvement is usually present, with large paraspinal

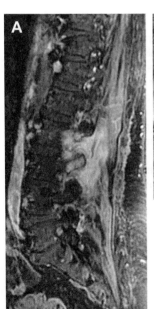
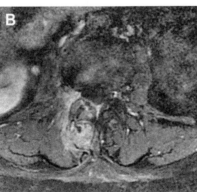

Fig. 9. Right L2-L3 facet joint septic arthritis. Fat-suppressed contrast-enhanced T1-weighted images (*A, B*) showed diffuse enhancement of the joint capsule, adjacent soft tissues, and contiguous osseous structures, such as pedicles and posterior vertebral elements.

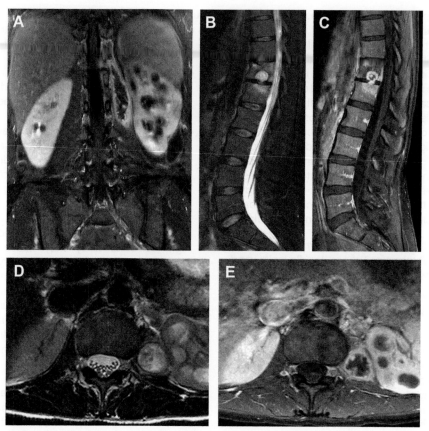

Fig. 10. A case of renal tuberculosis with left kidney enlargement (*A*) and intrarenal abscesses, contiguous spread to the left psoas muscle, involved by an abscess (*D, E*), and spondylodiskitis at T12-L1, with evidence of a T12 vertebral body intraosseous abscess (*B, C*).

abscesses, characterized by thin and smooth rim enhancement. The soft tissue masses typically calcify (**Figs. 11** and **12**). Meningeal involvement is common.

- Posterior elements can be involved.
- Anterior subligamentous spread can be more extensive than vertebral body involvement.

Brucella[31]

- The favorite location is the lower lumbar spine, typically isolated.
- Vertebral body is typically relatively preserved.
- Disk involvement is present and predominant.
- Paraspinal/epidural space involvement is typically not present.
- Posterior elements are typically not involved.
- Anterior subligamentous spread is uncommon.
- Brucellar spondylitis may also show imaging features of radiculitis, arachnoiditis, and neuritis. Especially in lumbar brucellosis, the peritoneum adjacent to the involved vertebra may be thickened and periaortic lymph nodes may be enlarged.

Fungi[32]

- The favorite location is the lumbar spine with multilevel involvement and presence of skip lesions.
- Vertebral body involvement is variable, usually without severe vertebral destruction.
- The disk is typically spared with only faint or absent signal abnormalities and preservation of the internuclear cleft.
- Paraspinal/epidural space involvement is present with small paraspinal abscesses with thick and irregular rim enhancement. The contrast enhancement may be mild or absent, because of the poor inflammatory reaction of immunocompromised patients.
- Involvement of posterior elements and rib heads is possible.
- Anterior subligamentous spread is common, such as in the tubercular form.

Role of Interventional Radiology in the Diagnosis: Image-Guided Biopsy

An image-guided biopsy is recommended in patients with suspected SD based on clinical,

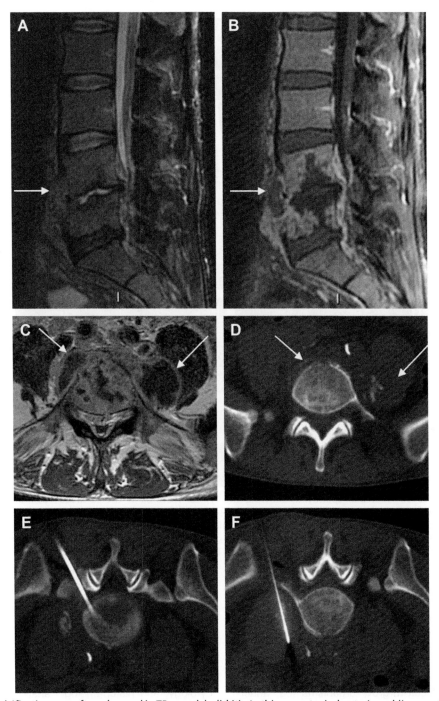

Fig. 11. Calcifications are often observed in TB spondylodiskitis. In this case a typical anterior subligamentous abscess was seen at L4-L5 on sagittal fat-suppressed T2-weighted (*arrow* on *A*) and contrast-enhanced fat-suppressed T1-weighted (*arrow* on *B*). The axial contrast-enhanced T1-weighted image (*C*) showed perivertebral fluid collections on the left abutting the psoas muscle (*arrows* on *C*), and the unenhanced CT (*D*) depicted granular and clumped calcifications within the collections (*arrows* on *D*). The CT-guided biopsy targeted the disk space (*E*) and the largest fluid collection (*F*).

laboratory, and imaging studies, when a microbiologic diagnosis has not been established by blood cultures or serologic tests.[33] In patients with sepsis, or presence of an abscess with neurologic

compromise, immediate surgical intervention and initiation of an empiric antimicrobial therapy is recommended.[33,34] If a polymicrobial osteomyelitis is suspected, a biopsy should be performed

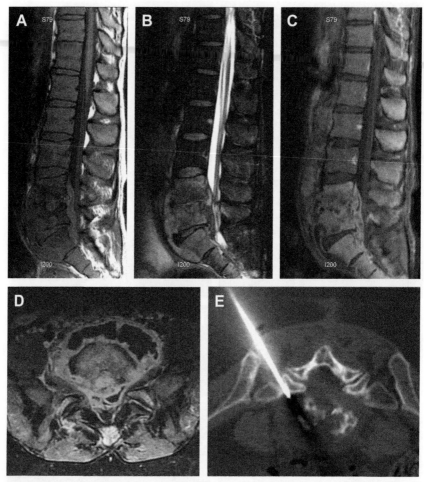

Fig. 12. A case of tubercular spondylitis showing the typical features of the so-called "ossifluent abscess," with multilevel L4-S1 involvement, subligamentous abscess along the anterior aspect of the L4-S1 vertebral bodies, intraosseous abscesses in L4 and L5 vertebral bodies, relative sparing of the disk space L5-S1, and epidural abscess (*A–D*). A pigtail drainage was inserted in the subligamentous abscess through a diskal access under CT-guidance (*E*) and left in place for a few days to help healing.

regardless of whether the blood cultures are positive.[35] The biopsy sensitivity is superior to blood culture sensitivity (77% [range, 47%–100%] vs 58% [range, 30%–78%][4] when both are performed before antibiotic therapy[33]). In patients with a nondiagnostic first image-guided biopsy, further biopsy sampling should be performed to exclude difficult-to-grow organisms (eg, anaerobes, fungi, *Brucella* species, or mycobacteria).[34] An image-guided biopsy has to be repeated if the first biopsy is negative or grows skin contaminants and surgical biopsy should be warranted if image-guided biopsies are negative.[33] Biopsy has been described to lead to a change in management in 35% of cases.[36] The amount of harvested material is relevant because fine-needle aspirate has low yield compared with core biopsy samples.[33,37–40] The target for biopsy

should be the focus of active abnormal contrast enhancement and should include disk material, subchondral bone, and aspirate of extravertebral collections, when present. Sample must be submitted for microbiology test (aerobes, anaerobes, fungi; mycobacterium and brucella in patients with a suggestive history and in endemic areas), cytology, and histopathologic analysis, because the presence of white blood cells allows one to distinguish infection from contamination, and the presence of granulomas suggest tuberculosis or brucellosis. If the antibiotic treatment has already been started, a 48-hour antibiotic-free interval allows a better yield. A longer free time interval would allow better yield but it has to be balanced with clinical risks.[33]

The percutaneous biopsy, feasible from the upper cervical spine to the sacrum and coccyx, can be performed under fluoroscopic guidance or CT guidance, mainly depending on local anatomy, availability, and operator preferences. Thorough knowledge of fluoroscopic landmarks is required when using fluoroscopy.[41] When using CT it may be useful to tilt the CT gantry to conform to the different axis of spine accesses.[42] We recommend the use of coaxial biopsy systems, which allow one to perform multiple sampling passes. A large-bore (from 14 to 8 G) access cannula is first placed at the periphery of the area to be sampled, and coaxially, multiple core samples and aspirates are performed with a biopsy cannula, under vacuum suction (**Fig. 13**). The biopsy can be performed as an outpatient procedure, under local anesthesia or conscious sedation, whereas general anesthesia is preferred for cervical spine access. For thoracolumbar biopsies, the access cannula can be directed to the disk space, with a posterolateral paravertebral approach, passing dorsal and medial to the nerve root in the foramen. Through the access needle the biopsy cannula can be advanced to sample the disk space, and then be retracted and redirected caudally toward the disk end plate, for sampling of the cartilage and subchondral bone; alternatively a curved coaxial biopsy cannula can be used to obtain samples from different regions of the lesion. An alternative, safe, and effective way to perform biopsy in case of suspected SD is through a steeply oblique caudocranial transpedicular approach, which through incremental coaxial advancement of the biopsy cannula allows one to sample material from the inferior disk end plate first, then from the disk space, and finally from the superior disk end plate (**Fig. 14**).[43] Cervical disk biopsies are performed with an anterolateral approach, passing between the neurovascular bundle and the trachea, for disks between C3-C4 and C7-T1, whereas a subzygomatic transmaxillary approach can be performed to sample the upper cervical spine.[41]

Role of Imaging in the Follow-Up

Follow-up imaging is not recommended when a favorable clinical and laboratory evolution of SD is present. If a clinical assessment at 4 weeks demonstrates a persistency of fever, pain, or elevated CRP level, imaging is indicated in the suspicion of treatment failure.[33] If an epidural abscess is suspected based on increasing back pain or new neurologic symptoms, imaging with MR imaging is indicated. MR imaging is also required to demonstrate the resolution of large

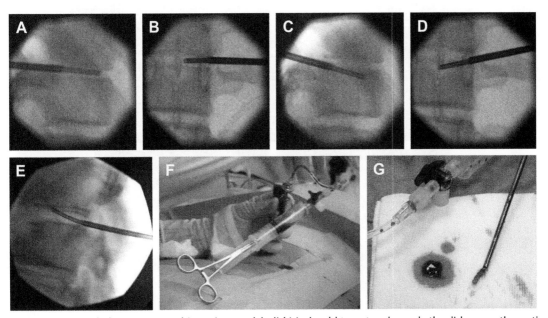

Fig. 13. Image-guided percutaneous biopsy in spondylodiskitis should target and sample the disk space, the cartilage, and the subchondral bone of adjacent disk end plates. In these examples fluoroscopic-guidance is used. With a coaxial system the access cannula is brought to the posterior margin of the disk space with a posterolateral approach; coaxially a biopsy cannula is advanced to sample the disk space (*A, B*), then the cannula is retracted, redirected caudally, and advanced again to sample the subchondral bone (*C, D*). Multiple coaxial biopsy passes can be performed with a curved cannula to obtain sampling from different areas of the lesion (*E*). The biopsy is performed under vacuum suction (*F*), and solid tissue core samples and fluid material are obtained (*G*), to be sent to microbiology and pathology examination.

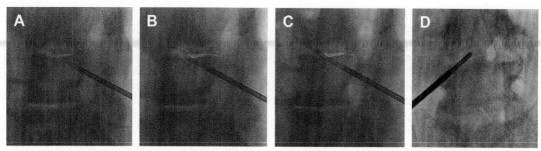

Fig. 14. Modified fluoroscopically guided steeply oblique transpedicular approach to obtain biopsy from the subchondral bone (*A*), disk space (*B*), and opposed disk end plate (*C*). The anteroposterior view (*D*) is used to confirm access direction toward midline, at the center of the disk space.

abscesses that have not been surgically treated before discontinuing antibiotic therapy.

The correlation between MR imaging findings and healing is poor.[44] Indeed, MR imaging findings, such as disk space enhancement, bone marrow edema, and vertebral enhancement, may persist or even worsen during treatment. Diminished paravertebral soft tissue swelling is reported

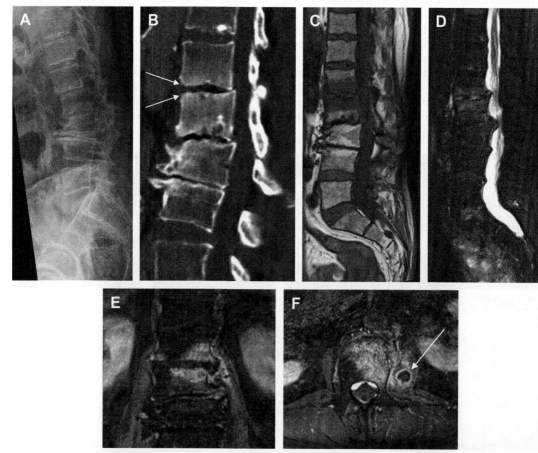

Fig. 15. A patient with chronic low back pain presented with recently worsened back tenderness and malaise. Plain films (*A*) and CT (*B*) showed severe multilevel degenerative disk pathology, with disk space narrowing, vacuum disk, osteophytosis, and end plates sclerosis. MR imaging (*C–F*) revealed edema in the L1-L2 disk and adjacent subchondral regions on T1-weighted (*C*) and STIR (*D*) images, with contrast enhancement on fat-suppressed enhanced T1-weighted images (*E, F*). These findings could still be compatible with degenerative Modic I changes, but on axial enhanced image a small abscess was visible in the left psoas muscle (*arrow* on *F*), which is highly specific for an infectious process. Retrospectively cortical erosion at the insertion site of the anulus fibrosus was visible on CT at L1-L2 (*arrows* on *B*), as an early CT sign of spondylodiskitis.

as the first signs of improvement.[45] Another sign of healing is the evidence of high-signal-intensity rim on the T1-weighted image at the edge of the lesion and the evidence of reconstituted marrow that appears predominantly fatty with higher signal intensity than normal marrow on T1 and T2. Follow-up MR imaging often demonstrates vertebral body height loss. In contrast, lower signal of the bone marrow on T1- and T2-weighted images may be a reflection of reactive sclerosis and fibrosis caused by healing.

It is recommended that radiography should be carried out once treatment is completed to assess spinal deformity.

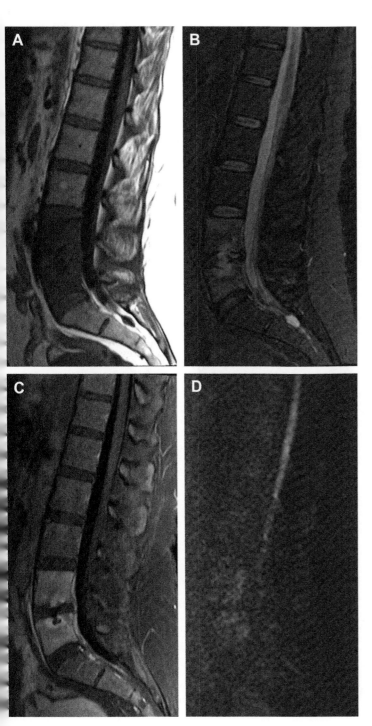

Fig. 16. DWI. MR imaging with sagittal T1-weighted (*A*), fat-suppressed T2-weighted (*B*), fat-suppressed contrast-enhanced T1-weighted (*C*), and b700 DWI (*D*) images, showing diffuse bone marrow edema of the L4 and L5 vertebral bodies, focal enhancing irregularities along the disk end plates. On DWI images there was hyperintense signal of the affected vertebral bodies, without claw sign, reinforcing the suspicion of infectious spondylodiskitis rather than degenerative Modic I changes.

WHAT THE REFERRING PHYSICIAN NEEDS TO KNOW

Among the conditions that may resemble SD, the differential diagnosis in the adult population is mainly with Modic type 1 degenerative end plate changes and erosive intervertebral osteochondrosis. In children chronic recurrent multifocal osteomyelitis has to be taken into account.[46]

- Modic type I degenerative end plate changes may resemble early pyogenic SD. Key differential findings are the signal intensity of the disk that shows less T2 hyperintensity or low T2 signal with only mild linear enhancement after contrast. There might be some adjacent soft tissue involvement, but never with fluid collections and abscesses. There are signal changes of the adjacent vertebral bodies related to edema but the cortical continuity of the vertebral end plate is generally respected. The identification on DWI of a well-marginated, linear, and

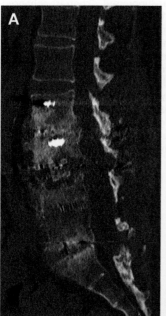
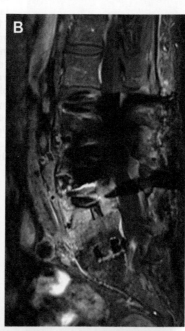
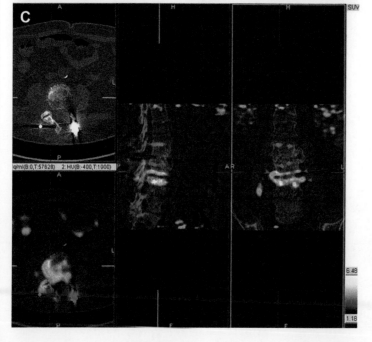

Fig. 17. PET-CT can serve as a problem solving imaging tool in selected cases. This patient with lumbar multilevel hardware stabilization presented with worsening resistant back pain and marked inflammatory syndrome. CT (A) showed nonspecific disk space abnormalities, such as narrowing, end plates irregularities, sclerosis, and resorption, at multiple levels; MR imaging (B) was largely obscured by metallic artefacts and uneven fat suppression, with contrast enhancement of the L4 vertebral body. PET-CT combined the relative insensitivity of CT to hardware metallic artefacts with the specificity of MR imaging, showing increased focal metabolic activity along the end plates at L3-L4 (C), strongly suggestive of infectious process.

typically paired region of high signal within the adjoined involved vertebral bodies at the boundaries between the normal bone marrow and vascularized bone marrow, the so-called "claw sign," suggests Modic type I degenerative end plate changes (**Figs. 15–17**).[21]

- Erosive intervertebral osteochondrosis is the destructive form of intervertebral osteochondrosis with inflammatory degeneration of the intervertebral disk. It is characterized by T2 hypersignal of the disk with gadolinium enhancement, in addition to the characteristic changes of Modic I. Compared with SD, edema of the vertebral bone marrow adjacent to the disk space uncommonly reaches the middle part and almost never extends to the opposite end plate. Erosion of the adjacent end plates occurs with no major destruction. No paravertebral/epidural involvement occurs. There is minimal or no osteophytosis. Dense sclerosis with bone erosions can be seen.
- Dialysis-related spondyloarthropathy is related to amyloid deposition in the disk and ligamentum flavum in patients with history of dialysis. Decrease of disk height and erosion of the subchondral bone mimic SD. However, on MR imaging, the T2 appears hypointense because of amyloid deposition, with a signal intensity similar to that of muscle (**Fig. 18**). The most commonly involved area is the lower cervical spine. Posterior element involvement is present and this also helps the differential diagnosis with SD.
- Chronic recurrent multifocal osteomyelitis is a nonbacterial osteomyelitis, an autoinflammatory disorder that mostly affects children, characterized by periodic bone pain, fever, and the appearance of multiple bone lesions involving the metaphyseal area of long bones, the clavicle, the shoulder, and any other bone location including the spine. Skeletal manifestations may be synchronous or metachronous with a relapsing remitting course. The lesions resemble infectious SD and are lytic and destructive in the early phase, and sclerotic and reactive in the late phase (**Fig. 19**). The treatment is based on nonsteroidal antiinflammatory drugs, bisphosphates, and steroids.

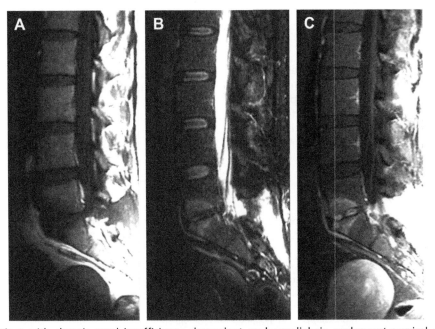

Fig. 18. Patient with chronic renal insufficiency, dependent on hemodialysis, underwent surgical discectomy 4 years before, now being investigated for 6-week history of low back pain. MR imaging with sagittal T1-weighted (*A*), STIR (*B*), and fat-suppressed contrast-enhanced T1-weighted (*C*) images shows abnormal signal, related to edema and inflammation in the L5-S1 disk and adjacent end plates. No fluid collections are noted. Although the findings are indistinguishable from spondylodiskitis in the early phase, the clinical diagnosis of hemodialysis-related spondyloarthropathy was made. The changes completely resolved with anti-inflammatory therapy, without use of antibiotics. (*Courtesy of* Prof. A. Leone, MD, Rome, Italy.)

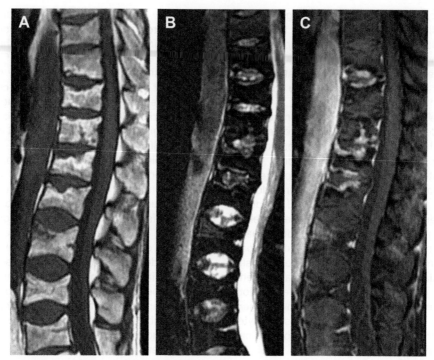

Fig. 19. Adolescent patient with multifocal migrating localizations of noninfectious osteomyelitis, diagnosed as chronic recurrent multifocal osteomyelitis. MR imaging with sagittal T1-weighted (*A*), STIR (*B*), and fat-suppressed contrast-enhanced T1-weighted (*C*) images shows multilevel inflammatory changes along disk end plates, with edema and contrast enhancement, and wedge deformity of vertebral bodies. Similar changes were also present at other skeletal sites. (*Courtesy of* Prof. A. Leone, MD, Rome, Italy.)

SUMMARY

Imaging plays a key role in the management of SD. MR imaging can contribute early in the diagnosis by detecting edema and contrast uptake of the vertebral end plates and intervertebral disk. Image-guided percutaneous biopsy is crucial in the identification of the causative agent to address the appropriate antimicrobial therapy.

REFERENCES

1. Duarte RM, Vaccaro AR. Spinal infection: state of the art and management algorithm. Eur Spine J 2013; 22(12):2787–99.
2. Fantoni M, Trecarichi EM, Rossi B, et al. Epidemiological and clinical features of pyogenic spondylodiscitis. Eur Rev Med Pharmacol Sci 2012; 16(Suppl 2):2–7.
3. Silber JS, Anderson DG, Vaccaro AR, et al. Management of postprocedural discitis. Spine J 2002;2(4): 279–87.
4. Mylona E, Samarkos M, Kakalou E, et al. Pyogenic vertebral osteomyelitis: a systematic review of clinical characteristics. Semin Arthritis Rheum 2009; 39(1):10–7.
5. Gouliouris T, Aliyu SH, Brown NM. Spondylodiscitis: update on diagnosis and management. J Antimicrob Chemother 2010;65(Suppl 3):11–24.
6. Sobottke R, Seifert H, Fätkenheuer G, et al. Current diagnosis and treatment of spondylodiscitis. Dtsch Arztebl Int 2008;105(10):181–7.
7. Turunc T, Demiroglu YZ, Uncu H, et al. A comparative analysis of tuberculous, brucellar and pyogenic spontaneous spondylodiscitis patients. J Infect 2007;55(2):158–63.
8. Priest DH, Peacock JEJ. Hematogenous vertebral osteomyelitis due to *Staphylococcus aureus* in the adult: clinical features and therapeutic outcomes. South Med J 2005;98(9):854–62.
9. Tsiodras S, Falagas ME. Clinical assessment and medical treatment of spine infections. Clin Orthop Relat Res 2006;444:38–50.
10. Fucs PM, Meves R, Yamada HH. Spinal infections in children: a review. Int Orthop 2012; 36(2):387–95.
11. Khan MH, Smith PN, Rao N, et al. Serum C-reactive protein levels correlate with clinical response in patients treated with antibiotics for wound infections after spinal surgery. Spine J 2006;6(3):311–5.
12. Hopkinson N, Stevenson J, Benjamin S. A case ascertainment study of septic discitis: clinical,

microbiological and radiological features. QJM 2001;94(9):465–70.

13. Ratcliffe JF. Anatomic basis for the pathogenesis and radiologic features of vertebral osteomyelitis and its differentiation from childhood discitis. A microarteriographic investigation. Acta Radiol Diagn (Stockh) 1985;26(2):137–43.

14. Arizono T, Oga M, Shiota E, et al. Differentiation of vertebral osteomyelitis and tuberculous spondylitis by magnetic resonance imaging. Int Orthop 1995; 19(5):319–22.

15. Henriques CQ. Osteomyelitis as a complication in urology; with special reference to the paravertebral venous plexus. Br J Surg 1958;46(195): 19–28.

16. Babinchak TJ, Riley DK, Rotheram EBJ. Pyogenic vertebral osteomyelitis of the posterior elements. Clin Infect Dis 1997;25(2):221–4.

17. Varma R, Lander P, Assaf A. Imaging of pyogenic infectious spondylodiskitis. Radiol Clin North Am 2001;39(2):203–13.

18. Modic MT, Feiglin DH, Piraino DW, et al. Vertebral osteomyelitis: assessment using MR. Radiology 1985;157(1):157–66.

19. Colosimo C, Cianfoni A, Di Lella GM, et al. Contrast-enhanced MR imaging of the spine: when, why and how? How to optimize contrast protocols in MR imaging of the spine. Neuroradiology 2006; 48(Suppl 1):18–33.

20. Oztekin O, Calli C, Kitis O, et al. Reliability of diffusion weighted MR imaging in differentiating degenerative and infectious end plate changes. Radiol Oncol 2010;44(2):97–102.

21. Patel KB, Poplawski MM, Pawha PS, et al. Diffusion-weighted MRI "claw sign" improves differentiation of infectious from degenerative Modic type 1 signal changes of the spine. AJNR Am J Neuroradiol 2014;35(8):1647–52.

22. Love C, Patel M, Lonner BS, et al. Diagnosing spinal osteomyelitis: a comparison of bone and Ga-67 scintigraphy and magnetic resonance imaging. Clin Nucl Med 2000;25(12):963–77.

23. Gemmel F, Rijk PC, Collins JMP, et al. Expanding role of 18F-fluoro-D-deoxyglucose PET and PET/CT in spinal infections. Eur Spine J 2010; 19(4):540–51.

24. Aguila LA, Piraino DW, Modic MT, et al. The intranuclear cleft of the intervertebral disk: magnetic resonance imaging. Radiology 1985;155(1): 155–8.

25. Eastwood JD, Vollmer RT, Provenzale JM. Diffusion-weighted imaging in a patient with vertebral and epidural abscesses. AJNR Am J Neuroradiol 2002; 23(3):496–8.

26. Tali ET, Oner AY, Koc AM. Pyogenic spinal infections. Neuroimaging Clin N Am 2015;25(2): 193–208.

27. Hong SH, Kim SM, Ahn JM, et al. Tuberculous versus pyogenic arthritis: MR imaging evaluation. Radiology 2001;218(3):848–53.

28. Gouliamos AD, Kehagias DT, Lahanis S, et al. MR imaging of tuberculous vertebral osteomyelitis: pictorial review. Eur Radiol 2001;11(4):575–9.

29. Jung N-Y, Jee W-H, Ha K-Y, et al. Discrimination of tuberculous spondylitis from pyogenic spondylitis on MRI. AJR Am J Roentgenol 2004;182(6): 1405–10.

30. Moorthy S, Prabhu NK. Spectrum of MR imaging findings in spinal tuberculosis. AJR Am J Roentgenol 2002;179(4):979–83.

31. Ozaksoy D, Yucesoy K, Yucesoy M, et al. Brucellar spondylitis: MRI findings. Eur Spine J 2001;10(6): 529–33.

32. Williams RL, Fukui MB, Meltzer CC, et al. Fungal spinal osteomyelitis in the immunocompromised patient: MR findings in three cases. AJNR Am J Neuroradiol 1999;20(3):381–5.

33. Zimmerli W. Vertebral Osteomyelitis. N Engl J Med 2010;362:1022–9.

34. Berbari EF, Kanj SS, Kowalski TJ, et al. 2015 Infectious Diseases Society of America (IDSA) clinical practice guidelines for the diagnosis and treatment of native vertebral osteomyelitis in adults. Clin Infect Dis 2015;61(6):e26–46.

35. Patzakis MJ, Rao S, Wilkins J, et al. Analysis of 61 cases of vertebral osteomyelitis. Clin Orthop Relat Res 1991;264:178–83.

36. Rankine JJ, Barron DA, Robinson P, et al. Therapeutic impact of percutaneous spinal biopsy in spinal infection. Postgrad Med J 2004;80(948): 607–9.

37. Phadke DM, Lucas DR, Madan S. Fine-needle aspiration biopsy of vertebral and intervertebral disc lesions: specimen adequacy, diagnostic utility, and pitfalls. Arch Pathol Lab Med 2001; 125(11):1463–8.

38. Lucio E, Adesokan A, Hadjipavlou AG, et al. Pyogenic spondylodiskitis: a radiologic/pathologic and culture correlation study. Arch Pathol Lab Med 2000;124(5):712–6.

39. Chew FS, Kline MJ. Diagnostic yield of CT-guided percutaneous aspiration procedures in suspected spontaneous infectious diskitis. Radiology 2001; 218(1):211–4.

40. Michel SCA, Pfirrmann CWA, Boos N, et al. CT-guided core biopsy of subchondral bone and intervertebral space in suspected spondylodiskitis. AJR Am J Roentgenol 2006;186(4):977–80.

41. Massari F, Rumboldt Z, Vandergrift W, et al. Percutaneous image-guided C-spine procedures. Neurographics 2014;4(2):62–77.

42. Boulter DJ, Rumboldt Z, Bonaldi G, et al. Tilting the gantry for CT-guided spine procedures. Radiol Med 2014;119(10):750–7.

43. Layton KF, Thielen KR, Wald JT. A modified vertebro-plasty approach for spine biopsies. AJNR Am J Neuroradiol 2006;27(3):596–7.

44. Kowalski TJ, Layton KF, Berbari EF, et al. Follow-up MR imaging in patients with pyogenic spine infections: lack of correlation with clinical features. AJNR Am J Neuroradiol 2007;28(4):693–9.

45. Gillams AR, Chaddha B, Carter AP. MR appearances of the temporal evolution and resolution of infectious spondylitis. Am J Roentgenol 1996; 166(4):903–7.

46. Hong SH, Choi J-Y, Lee JW, et al. MR imaging assessment of the spine: infection or an imitation? Radiographics 2009;29(2):599–612.

Neuroimaging of the Postoperative Spine

Matteo Bellini, MD[a],*, Marco Ferrara, MD[a], Irene Grazzini, MD[b], Alfonso Cerase, MD[a]

KEYWORDS

- Magnetic resonance imaging • Postoperative spine • Spinal implants • Spinal surgery
- Spinal mini-invasive procedures

KEY POINTS

- Imaging of the postoperative spine is a challenging task for the radiologist and requires a general knowledge of the surgical and the new minimally invasive procedures, and of the evolving spinal instrumentation.
- Thanks to its capabilities, MR imaging is crucial for the evaluation of patients with recurrent or new symptoms after surgery or minimally invasive techniques, including both early and late complications.
- Technical aspects have to be considered to reduce artifacts from metallic devices.
- For the correct interpretation of the postoperative spinal imaging, the radiologist must have detailed understanding of the initial pathologic condition, the surgical procedure performed, the clinical presentation of the patient, the time interval from the procedure to the imaging study, and the evolution of the expected postoperative changes.

DISCUSSION OF PROBLEM/CLINICAL PRESENTATION

Neuroimaging following operative treatments of the spine, either by surgery or by minimally invasive procedures, depends on many factors, including cause of intervention, used technique, current symptoms, and time elapsed since procedure.[1–3] Generally, postoperative neuroimaging is performed in patients with clinical symptoms (mostly pain with or without neurologic deficit), in which minor and major complications are to be excluded.

Postoperative complications may occur after both surgery and minimally invasive procedures.[4] To understand the postoperative spinal neuroimaging, radiologists must know the operative and instrumentation options to explore the postprocedural complications.

SPINAL TREATMENT PROCEDURES IN PILLS AND NEW TRENDS

Classically, spinal treatments can be categorized as follows:

a. Decompressive, performed to remove herniated disc material or to relieve a segment of spinal stenosis.
b. Spinal stabilization/fusion procedures, in cases of spinal instability from degenerative disc disease, spondylolisthesis, trauma, tumors, infections, and iatrogenic causes, such as prior surgery.
c. A combination of both.

The authors have nothing to disclose.
[a] Neuroimaging and Neurointerventional Unit, Department of Neurological and Neurosensorial Sciences, General Hospital "Santa Maria Alle Scotte", Viale Bracci 16, Siena 53100, Italy; [b] Section of Radiological Sciences, Department of Medical, Surgical and NeuroSciences, University of Siena, Viale Bracci 16, Siena 53100, Italy
* Corresponding author. UOC NINT Neuroimmagini e Neurointerventistica, Azienda Ospedaliera Universitaria Senese, Viale Bracci n.16, Siena 53100, Italy.
E-mail addresses: matteo.bellini@ao-siena.toscana.it; matteo.bellini@icloud.com

mri.theclinics.com

Surgery

Spine surgery is used to treat diseases and injuries affecting the spinal column, including degenerative disorders, trauma, instability, deformities, infections, and tumors.

Surgical decompressive procedures include discectomy, laminotomy, laminectomy, and facetectomy. The term laminotomy refers to removal of only the inferior margin of the lamina and is often used in cases of microdiscectomy. In unilateral laminectomy, the entire lamina on one side of the spinous process is removed. Total or bilateral laminectomy involves removal of the lamina on both sides, plus the spinous process.

Surgical fusion procedures are often categorized based on the direction from which the spine is approached (anterior, posterior, lateral, caudal) as well as on their degree of invasiveness.[5–7] Surgical approaches are presented in Table 1.

Endoscopic Surgery

Endoscopic operations are now considered standard for intraforaminal/extraforaminal disc herniations.[8] The most common full endoscopic technique for patients with lumbar disc afflictions is the posterolateral *transforaminal* approach, but also full endoscopic *interlaminar* access was developed. Laser and bipolar radiofrequency current can be used. Basically, the transforaminal procedure has more limitations than the interlaminar, but it is less traumatic for the tissue.

Table 1
Surgical spine approaches

Type	Features
Cervical spine approaches	
Anterior cervical approaches	
Transoral-transpharyngeal approach	Access to anterior clivus, C1 and C2
Anteromedial approach	Complications can be spinal cord and, rarely, vascular injury
Posterior cervical approaches	
Laminotomy, laminectomy, laminoplasty	Degenerative spondylosis, disc herniations Complications are vertebral artery injury, post-laminectomy kyphosis, and new cervical radiculopathy
Posterior fusion hardware	Posterior cervical fusion typically involves lateral mass screws from C3 to C6, with traditional pedicle screws being reserved for the larger C2 and C7 levels
Thoracic approaches	Relatively high incidence of neurologic injury
Posterior and posterolateral approach	Transpedicular, transfacet, and transforaminal
Costotransversectomy	—
Lateral extracavitary approach	—
Lumbar approaches	
Anterior lumbar approach	Performed when posterior decompression is not required; vascular complications are reported less than 5%
Posterior lumbar approach	
Standard open discectomy	Laminotomy or hemilaminectomy, resection of the ligamentum flavum and retraction of neural elements
Posterior lumbar interbody fusion (PLIF)	Involves bilateral laminectomies and partial facetectomy
Transforaminal lumbar interbody fusion	Variation of PLIF through the foramen
Posterolateral fusion	Alternative or supplement to PLIF: bone graft is placed laterally between the transverse processes
Total disc replacement	Alternative to spinal fusion. Used for discogenic pain without significant spondylolisthesis

The combination of new operative accesses with technical advances now enables a full endoscopic procedure with visual control, which is considered equal to conventional operations when the indication criteria are heeded.

Indications for endoscopic surgery include the following:

- Sequestered or nonsequestered lumbar disc herniations, independent of localization;
- Recurrent disc herniations after conventional or full endoscopic operations;
- Lateral bony and ligamentary spinal canal stenoses;
- In selected cases, cysts of the zygapophyseal joint;
- In selected cases, positioning of implants in the intervertebral space;
- In selected cases, intervertebral debridement in spondylodiscitis.

Minimally Invasive Procedures: a Quick Look

In recent years, minimally invasive and/or less-invasive spine surgery and nonfusion devices have been developed. Minimally invasive techniques can reduce tissue damage and its consequences.

Vertebroplasty and balloon kyphoplasty may be carried out by vertebral interventional radiologists, orthopedists, and neurosurgeons.

Vertebroplasty describes a percutaneous procedure that introduces bone graft or acrylic cement (cementoplasty) to mechanically augment weakened vertebral bodies. Polymethylmethacrylate (PMMA) is the acrylic most commonly used as a bone filler in the treatment of pathologic and nonpathologic vertebral compression fractures.[9]

In addition, cementoplasty can be used in combination with fusion techniques, because anchorage of pedicle screws can be improved with cement augmentation. Augmentation of the screw can be achieved using 2 different techniques: (1) cement insertion through cannulated pedicle screws with slots, or (2) vertebroplasty followed by insertion of the pedicle screw into the cement (either open or minimally invasive).

Balloon kyphoplasty describes a percutaneous procedure that introduces an expansive device within the vertebral body to create a cavity that can be filled by cement. The goal is to achieve reduction of the fracture without injuring the lateral margin of the vertebral body.[8,10] Recently, many variants of balloon kyphoplasty are introduced. New titanium or polyetheretherketone implants can be used to obtain vertebral augmentation and relevant high restoration of

vertebral body in combination with less amount of PMMA or biologic cement injection.

New Trends

Recent advances have led to a number of technical developments including the following:

- Spinal navigation
- Fluoroscopy
- Spinal implants
- Bone substitutes, stem cells, and growth factors
- Endoscopy
- Microscopy
- Neurophysiological monitoring
- Improved instruments and retractors
- High-frequency surgery.

NEURORADIOLOGICAL EVALUATION

Postoperative spinal imaging techniques include radiographs, computed tomography (CT), and magnetic resonance (MR) imaging. CT and MR imaging may be performed before and after contrast media injection. Generally, radiographs are not used in the diagnosis of early or late postoperative complications but only to check the positioning of the metallic implants.

Even though the role of CT in the postsurgical spine is marginal, it is useful to check correct positioning of metallic implants after instrumentation or fusion procedures, to show laminotomy/laminectomy defect, to evaluate postoperative spinal stenosis, and the result of the spinal stabilization, as well as acute hematoma or gas-filled collections.

Magnetic Resonance Imaging

The high spatial and contrast resolution of MR imaging allow for better evaluation of soft tissues, bone marrow, and intraspinal content. Thus, MR imaging is the modality of choice in cases in which postoperative complications are suspected. Patient positioning is reported in **Box 1**.

There is no established protocol for the study of the postoperative spine with MR imaging. A routine protocol including sagittal fast-turbo spin echo (F-TSE) T2-weighted and T1-weighted and short-tau inversion-recovery (STIR) images, axial T1- weighted and T2-weighted, would suffice in most cases.

In the sagittal plane, T1-weighted and T2-weighted images offer complementary information. On T2-weighted images, normal intervertebral discs are bright. When degeneration, water loss, and collagen deposition occur, T2 relaxation time shortens and the discs gradually become darker (ie, low-signal degenerative or "black-disc"

Box 1
Patient positioning for MR imaging

- Supine position, if possible feet first, to diminish claustrophobia

- Patient as parallel as possible to the long axis of the magnet bore, to minimize inadvertent oblique positioning and to reduce the distorting effects of any underlying scoliosis

- Center of the coil(s) at the center of the region of interest, and in turn to the center of the magnet bore

- Lumbo-sacral spine: some authors[5] propose to avoid a knee support, as this reduces the lumbar lordosis, and may lead to underestimation of the size and presence of disc herniation

---

disease). Sagittal and axial T2-weighted images are also excellent for showing the spinal cord and the nerve roots of the cauda equina. Central spinal canal stenosis and impressions on the thecal sac are most easily recognized.

T1-weighted, STIR, or fat-suppressed T2-weighted images are sensitive to many bone-marrow diseases.

The normal epidural fat in the spine is bright on T1-weighted images and contrasts well with the dural sac and the adjacent normal or pathologic intervertebral disc. This is why axial T1-weighted images should be performed in the lumbar region. T1-weighted images are also excellent to differentiate between osteophytes and soft disc material.

Three-dimensional (3D)-TSE sequences have been suggested for MR imaging myelography. However, single-shot wide-slab T2-weighted sequences with a very long echo time have been proposed, making it possible to obtain a very short time imaging for single different views by running the sequence in different orientations, eliminating postprocessing.

Administration of a gadolinium-based contrast medium is particularly useful in patients with suspicious infection or previous discectomy, as discussed later. In gadolinium-enhanced T1-weighted images, fat-suppression techniques are used to increase the conspicuity of gadolinium-enhancement.

Metallic implants may create magnetic susceptibility artifacts. Metals that are not superparamagnetic, such as titanium, produce primarily radiofrequency artifacts, which are less marked, but may still obscure the neural foramina in the presence of pedicular screws. Sequences have been developed to reduce artifacts,[11,12] but their

use may necessitate increased image acquisition time and may result in image distortion. The technical aspects to be considered for artifact reduction are presented in Box 2.

POSTOPERATIVE IMAGING AFTER SURGICAL DISCECTOMY/HERNIECTOMY: NORMAL VERSUS PATHOLOGIC

Immediate postoperative imaging, in the first 6 to 8 postsurgical weeks, must be carefully evaluated considering changes in bone and soft tissues in relation to type and extent of surgery and time since the operation.

In early unenhanced images, postdiscectomy changes may mimic a residual disc herniation because of disruption of the annulus fibrosus and epidural tissue edema. Granulation tissue and/or fibrosis may physiologically present with mild epidural mass effect and homogeneous gadolinium-enhancement.

Epidural/peridural fibrosis consists of scar tissue that causes adherence of neural elements to other structures.[13] Because scarring is part of the normal reparative mechanism of tissue after surgery, most patients with epidural fibrosis are asymptomatic. Fibrosis-induced pain may be due to irritation, compression, and traction of the fibrotic tissue on adjacent nerve structures.

The main differential diagnosis of epidural fibrosis is recurrent disc herniation.

Box 2
Artifacts reduction in postoperative magnetic resonance imaging

- Fast spin echo sequences are better than conventional spin echo (SE) sequences, and these latter are better than gradient echo sequences. The shortest echo time possible is recommended for metal artifact reduction in SE sequences.

- Short-tau inversion-recovery sequences should be used for fat suppression, as sequences based on selective fat-saturation pulses are associated with poor homogeneity.

- Increase bandwidth.

- Decrease voxel size.

- Adjust frequency-encoding direction: it should be parallel to the long axis of pedicle screw, as the artifact produced will be linear and parallel to the metal material.

- Use of chemical shift fat-suppression techniques.

- Multisequence imaging (MAVRIC, SEMAC).

Recurrent disc herniation is the most common complication after discectomy. It is defined as disc herniation at the level of prior surgery, and may be ipsilateral or contralateral to the previous herniation.[13]

The reported incidence of recurrent disc herniation after lumbar discectomy varies between 3% and 18%.[14,15] It is important to remember that residual disc herniation and epidural fibrosis are not certainly pathologic because extruded disc fragment can regress spontaneously mainly by phagocytosis and the minor dural sac deforming mass effect deriving from scar tissue usually diminishes within 6 months after intervention. However, deformity of the dural sac accompanying epidural scar is to be considered abnormal when observed 6 months or more after surgery.[5]

Differential diagnosis between recurrent disc herniation and peridural fibrosis is important: notably, epidural scar does not benefit from reoperation.[16]

The herniated disc tissues are usually isointense to the parent disc on T1-weighted images and isointense to hyperintense to the disc on T2-weighted images (**Fig. 1**). After gadolinium administration, the disc material shows no enhancement; however, peripheral enhancement may be observed because of the granulation or dilated tissue of the adjacent epidural plexus.

If there is homogeneous diffuse enhancement, peridural fibrosis should be suspected; however, recurrent disc herniation may show a variable amount of enhancement in delayed scans. This is the result of gadolinium diffusion from adjacent vascularized granulation tissues into the capacious extracellular spaces of the relatively avascular disc and thus simulate peridural fibrosis. It is, therefore, mandatory to scan the patient as soon as possible after the administration of contrast.

Teaching points
Major differentiating criteria between recurrent disc herniation and epidural fibrosis include[17,18] the following:
- Obliteration of the epidural fat by uniformly enhancing epidural fibrosis in the anterior, lateral, and posterior epidural space in epidural fibrosis (T1 high signal of normal epidural fat also contrasts well with postoperative epidural fibrosis, which is dark);
- Lack of early central gadolinium-enhancement in recurrent or residual disc herniation;
- Homogeneous gadolinium-enhancement pattern of scar tissue.

Furthermore, slight deformation of the thecal sac and gadolinium-enhancement of nerve roots,

defining aseptic radiculitis, are expected after surgery. They reflect transient sterile inflammation within the nerve root undergoing repair (see **Fig. 1**). However, differentiation between abnormal postoperative nerve roots enhancement and normal slight pial-root enhancement, remains challenging within 6 months after surgery, but in the late phase should be considered abnormal. In asymptomatic patients, also aseptic reactive vertebral endplates and posterior annulus enhancement can be seen between 6 and 18 months.

COMPLICATIONS AFTER DISCECTOMY/ HERNIECTOMY

For both postsurgical and post–minimally invasive procedures, we can distinguish early or late complications.[3]

In the acute postsurgical stage, it is important to exclude bleeding, infection, and pseudomeningoceles, which can cause neurologic deficits; in the late postsurgery period, recurrent disc herniation, arachnoiditis, radiculitis, and fibrosis may be causes of persisting pain. For the minimally invasive procedures group, persisting or recurrent back pain in early or late time from the procedure can be encountered.

Fluid Collections

Fluid collections are common, and could be symptomatic or represent an incidental findings; however, they require careful evaluation and management. They can be classified by the following locations:

- Intraspinal, that is, within the dural compartment;
- Paraspinal, that is anterior, lateral, or posterior the spinal axis (**Figs. 2** and **3**).

Fluid collections mainly include the following:

- Hematoma;
- Seroma;
- Pseudomeningocele;
- Abscess.

Hematoma
A spinal hematoma is a focal collection of blood of variable extent that can occur within or outside of the spinal canal. The incidence rate is estimated to be less than 1% of patients requiring spine surgery. It has been suggested that spinal epidural hematomas develop from a rupture of the internal vertebral venous plexus of Batson.

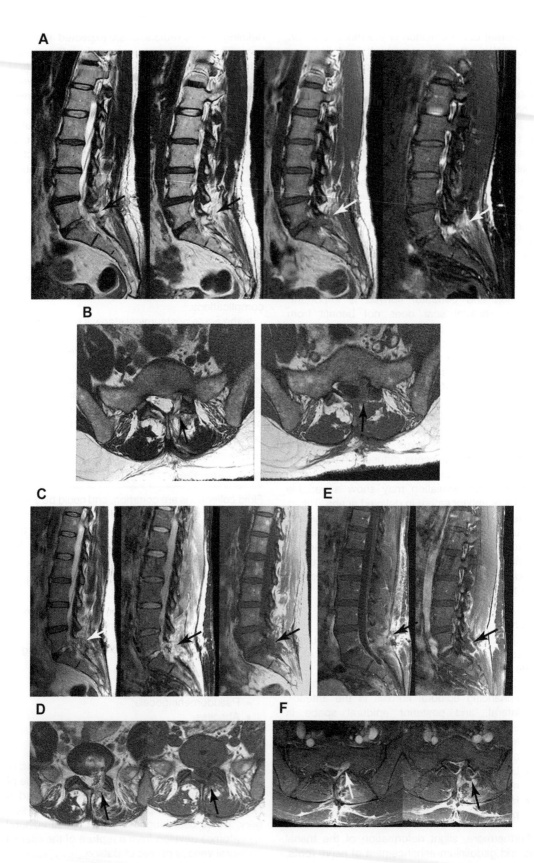

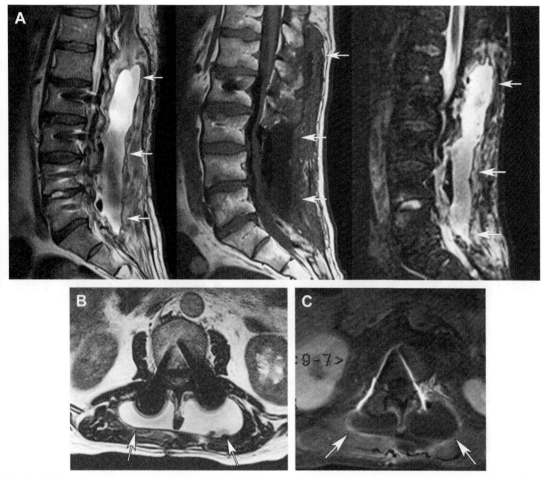

Fig. 2. A 60-year-old man 1 year after L3–L4 laminectomy and L1–S1 posterior stabilization. Sagittal T2-weighted, T1-weighted and STIR images (*A*) and axial T2-weighted (*B*) images show a large posterior fluid collection at the L1–S1 level (*arrows*). The collection is isointense with the CSF. An air-fluid level is seen inside the collection and in the epidural space (*C, arrows*).

Postoperative hemorrhage typically presents hours to days after surgery[5] (**Fig. 4**). MR imaging shows mixed blood breakdown products and is more sensitive than CT especially thanks to T2*-weighted images. MR imaging appearance of epidural hematoma is summarized in **Table 2**. Some hematomas may reach large sizes and can extend into the central spinal canal to compress the spinal nerves and/or spinal cord.[3] Spinal subdural hematomas are rare, with only a few cases of subacute presentation reported in the literature associated with surgical trauma.[19–21] The onset of a subdiaphragmatic hematoma has been described as a rare complication in the thoracoscopic approach for thoracic disc herniation.[22]

Fig. 1. A 30-year-old woman complaining of persistent left leg pain after surgery for disc herniation. Sagittal T2-weighted (*A*) and axial T1-weighted (*B*) images show postoperative recurrent disc herniation after hemilaminectomy; there is also a scar contacting the left S1 nerve root (*arrows*). The patient underwent surgical revision for scar removal. After surgery, she presented with worsening of the pain and left leg sensitive loss. Postsurgery sagittal T2-weighted (*C*) and T1-weighted axial (*D*) images show inhomogeneous inflammatory tissue encroaching the left S1 nerve root, associated with disc material along the surgical bed (*arrows*). Sagittal (*E*) and axial (*F*) contrast-enhanced T1-weighted images show reactive dural and left S1 nerve root enhancement consistent with sterile radiculitis (*arrows*). A small paravertebral fluid collection is seen at L5–S1 laminectomy (*black arrow* in F). There was no suspected infection and the patient was treated with steroid, with complete resolution of the symptoms.

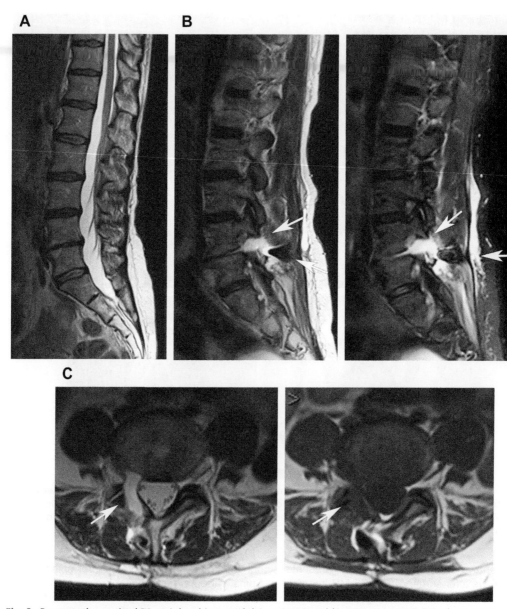

Fig. 3. Preoperative sagittal T2-weighted images (*A*) in a 51-year-old woman presenting with L4–L5 disc herniation. She underwent surgical discectomy. Postoperative sagittal T2-weighted and fat-suppressed contrast-enhanced images (*B*) and axial T2-weighted and T1-weighted images (*C*) show a right posterolateral epidural collection at the hemilaminectomy site, T1-hypointense and T2-hyperintense, compatible with seroma mildly compressing the thecal sac (*arrow*). Note an interspinous spacer (*B, lower arrow*). The fluid analysis was unremarkable.

In addition to the detection and guide for proper treatment, MR imaging is an essential tool also in the follow-up so as to evaluate eventual subinfection of the hematoma.

Seroma

Seroma is a lymphatic fluid collection resulting from damage to local lymphatic vessels: it may be surrounded by a fibrous capsule. It is rare, may be subcutaneous or in the paraspinal soft tissues, and often overlap with hematoma. At MRI, it shows fluid signal with low T1 and high T2 and DWI signal: a level can be noted in the collection, as well as a slight peripheral gadolinium-enhancement. Differential diagnosis include other postoperative paraspinal collections. Compression bandage and percutaneous and/or surgical drainage may be indicated when seroma is

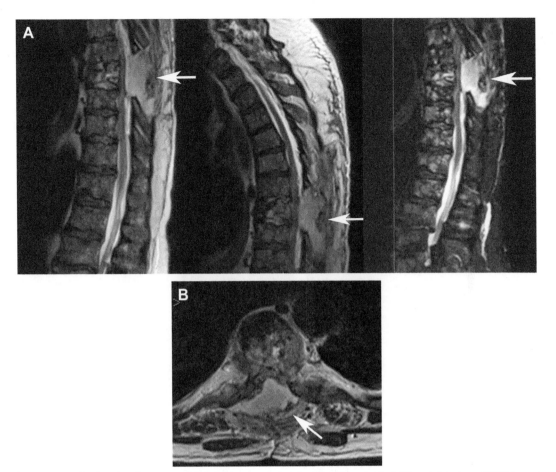

Fig. 4. Severe back pain after recent bilateral laminectomy. Sagittal T1-weighted, T2-weighted, and STIR images (*A*) and axial T2-weighted images (*B*) demonstrate a dorsal epidural and deep soft tissues fluid collection at D8 level, with encroachment on the spinal cord. The collection (*arrow*) is predominantly T1 hypo-isointense and T2-hyperintense and is consistent with a subacute hematoma.

large and symptomatic, or there is a possibility of infection.

Pseudomeningocele

Pseudomeningocele is a collection of cerebrospinal fluid (CSF) extending from the spinal canal into the adjacent paraspinal tissue. It is rare, although it has been reported in up to 2% of

patients undergoing lumbar laminectomy.[2,23] It typically develops after laceration of the dural sac or following incomplete closure of the dural sac during surgery.[5] The margin is composed of reactive fibrous tissue and not by meninges. This is in contrast with the true meningocele, congenital, and arachnoid-lined. Usually, a pseudomeningocele protrudes through a surgical

Table 2
Magnetic resonance appearance of hematoma

Stage	Age	Hemoglobin	Signal T1	Signal T2
Hyperacute	<12 h	Oxyhemoglobin	Isointense	Hyperintense
Acute	1–3 d	Deoxymethemoglobin	Hypointense	Hypointense
Early subacute	3–7 d	Intracellular methemoglobin	Hyperintense	Hypointense
Late subacute	7–14 d	Extracellular methemoglobin	Hyperintense	Hyperintense
Chronic	>2 wk	Hemosiderin	Hypointense	Hypointense

bony defect of the posterior spinal elements to form a cystic lesion with imaging characteristics comparable to CSF on ultrasound, CT, and MR imaging (**Fig. 5**). Notably, T2-weighted sequences in sagittal and axial planes are useful to visualize the collection and its communications/fistulae with the dural sac.[2] A fine peripheral contrast enhancement can be seen, but if more conspicuous it may raise the suspicion of superinfection.

Pseudomeningoceles are sometimes incidental findings on imaging. However, partly because of mass effect, they may also be responsible for low-back pain.

Teaching points
- Pseudomeningocele usually is contiguous with postsurgical type and shows CSF signal on MR imaging sequences.

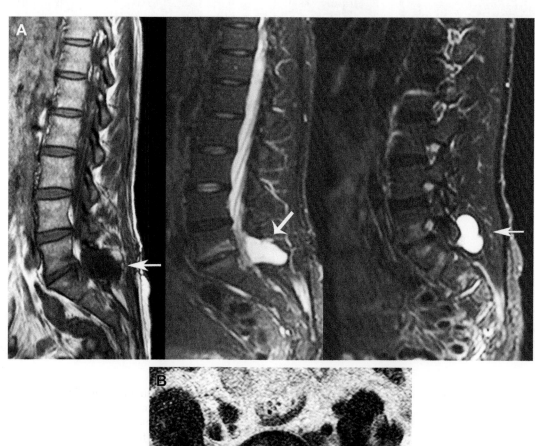

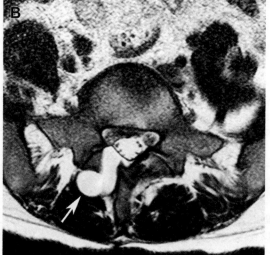

Fig. 5. A 40-year-old woman following L5–S1 hemilaminectomy for spinal canal decompression. T1-weighted, T2-weighted, and fat-suppressed sagittal (A), and T2-weighted axial (B) images show a fluid collection in the laminectomy bed at L5–S1 with mild mass effect on the posterior aspect of the thecal sac (arrow). Note also bone marrow changes (Modic I) in the vertebral body of L5 and S1, according to reactive edema.

- An intense enhancement raises suspicion for possible infection and abscess.

Abscess

Abscesses are circumscribed infected fluid collections. Intravenous antibiotic prophylaxis has decreased their incidence, which ranges from 0.2% to 20%.[23] The most common pathogen is *Staphylococcus aureus*, followed by *Staphylococcus epidermidis*, and *Propionibacterium acnes* in patients with implants.[24]

At MR imaging, the collection is irregular, hypointense on T1-weighted images, hyperintense on T2-weighted images and diffusion weighted images, with peripheral irregular prominent gadolinium-enhancement (**Fig. 6**), and low apparent diffusion coefficient.

An epidural abscess may cause neurologic symptoms due to spinal cord/nerve root compression. Imaging-guided needle aspiration, before the beginning of the antibiotic therapy, is considered to confirm the diagnosis and to determine the

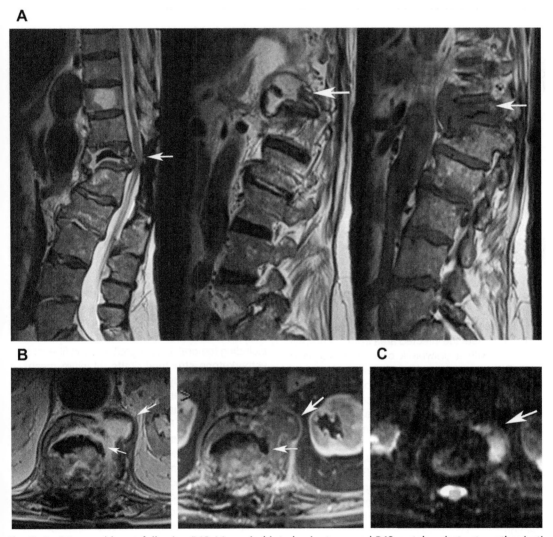

Fig. 6. An 84-year-old man following D12–L1 surgical interlaminotomy and D12 vertebroplasty at another institution. Sagittal T2-weighted and T1-weighted (*A*) images demonstrate space cement filling into D12 vertebral body (*arrow*), subsequent new compression fracture with posterior wall involvement, and spinal canal stenosis. The fluid collection (*arrow*) into the vertebral body and in the left paravertebral is T2-hyperintense and T1-hypointense. Axial T2-weighted and contrast-enhanced T1-weighted (*B*) sequences clarify the extent of the collection into the vertebral body and in the left paravertebral space (*arrows*) and show irregular peripheral enhancement. Diffusion-weighted imaging (*C*) shows restricted diffusion (*arrow*). Surgical exploration and drainage confirmed an abscess.

subsequent management, which may include medical therapy or drainage.[25]

SPONDYLODISCITIS

Spondylodiscitis is a serious complication, with a reported incidence of 0.2% to 2.75% after surgery,[26] but it can be encountered also after percutaneous disc treatment, as well as after diagnostic procedures, such as discography and myelography.[27] The infection is due to direct intraoperative contamination or to hematogenous seeding of the vertebral bodies. The main organisms involved are S epidermidis or S aureus.[28] Diagnosis depends on a combination of clinical, laboratory, and imaging findings. Symptoms are usually nonspecific: therefore, it should be suspected in patients with increased lumbar pain after procedures, unable to stand up, and abnormal laboratory tests.

The modality of choice is gadolinium-enhanced MR imaging with fat saturation, which allows for the evaluation of the bone edema and discitis earlier than other imaging techniques.[29] Characteristic findings include the following:

- Diminished disc height;
- Vertebral body and disc space decreased intensity on T1-weighted images;
- Increased signal intensity on T2-weighted imaging secondary to edema;
- Endplate definition loss.

These disc changes are accompanied by increased bone marrow intensity signaling due to edema (Fig. 7). Early in the infection process, STIR sequences offer higher signal intensity to help differentiate the infected area from the normal spine, but with a drawback of inferior anatomic detail. Diffusion-weighted imaging shows hyperintensity of the central necrotic region and hypointensity on the apparent diffusion coefficient map (restricted diffusion). MR imaging is also advantageous for evaluating the extension of the infections by visualizing at the same time the bone marrow, paravertebral soft tissues, spinal canal, and spinal nervous structures.[30] Rim-enhancing fluid collections, ascending epidural collections, evidence of bony destruction, and progressive bone marrow signal changes are suggestive of infection.[31]

Although diagnosing spondylodiscitis in the unoperated patient can be straightforward, it is more challenging after surgery. The operated level almost always shows changes due to the surgery itself and the postoperative aseptic inflammatory response. Peripheral gadolinium-enhancement of the remaining disk without adjacent reactive

endplate changes is suggestive of infections, whereas linear areas of enhancement are more likely postsurgical. Distinguishing between postsurgical changes and spondylodiscitis is crucial for the patient's management.

Postoperative spondylodiscitis

- An enhancing soft tissue mass surrounding the affected spinal level in the perivertebral and epidural spaces is highly suggestive of septic spondylodiscitis.
- Absence of peridiscal marrow changes (ie, low signal intensity on T1-weighted and high signal intensity on T2-weighted images) makes the diagnosis of septic spondylodiscitis unlikely.
- Absence of gadolinium-enhancement of the intervertebral disc space makes the diagnosis of septic spondylodiscitis unlikely.

If, in any case of suspected postoperative infection, MR imaging is not able to exclude or confirm septic spondylodiscitis, biopsy is recommended,[32] although it may result negative (Box 3).

POSTOPERATIVE IMAGING AFTER INTERVERTEBRAL FUSION AND INSTRUMENTATION

Spinal instrumentation techniques have expanded dramatically during the past decades. The goal of spinal instrumentation is to maintain the correct anatomic alignment of spinal segments. Various interbody device materials have been used, including femoral ring allograft, carbon fiber or polyetherketone structural grafts, titanium mesh, or threaded interbody cage constructs.[10]

Generally, materials used in orthopedic surgery can be classified into 3 groups: metals, ceramics, and polymers (ie, PMMA).[8]

Fixation devices are designed for the cervical, thoracic, lumbar, and sacral segments using anterior, posterior, transverse, videoarthroscopic, and combined approaches. In most cases, bone grafting with or without recombinant human bone morphogenetic protein is also performed[5,8,13,33,34] to fill defects, bridge defects, or to promote spondylodesis.

The main types of instrumentation are listed in Table 3.[6,35,36]

Device Imaging

Evaluation of the spine following placement of orthopedic hardware should include a description of

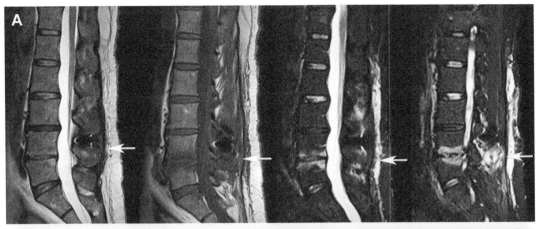

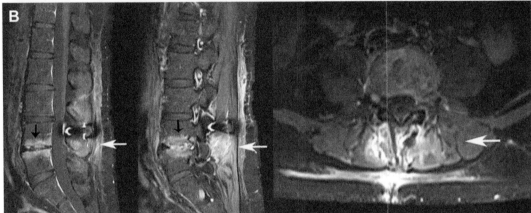

Fig. 7. Septic spondylodiscitis. The patient was 1 month after posterior fusion and stabilization with interspinous spacers. T2-weighted, T1-weighted, and STIR sagittal (*A*) images show diminished disc height, vertebral body and disc space, decreased T1-intensity and increased T2-intensity, and endplate definition loss, at the level indicated by *white arrows*. These disc changes are accompanied by increased bone marrow intensity signal due to edema. Sagittal and axial (*B*) T1 gadolinium-enhanced fat-suppressed images demonstrate disc and endplate enhancement (*black arrows*), as well as para-vertebral enhancement (*white arrows*).

Box 3
Causes of negative spine biopsy in postoperative spine
Concurrent antibiotic therapy
Insufficient sample
Lavage aspiration only
Sample of incorrect site
Incorrect sample handling

the type of hardware used and its location in the spine. The exact location is necessary to the surgeon to confirm the instrumentation was placed in the proper levels as planned before the procedure.

The main hardware-related complications include the following:

- Malpositioning
- Implant migration
- Loosening
- Implant fracture
- Superficial and deep infections
- Graft material herniation, anteriorly or posteriorly (depending on the approach used), which may cause neurologic compromise[6]

Reliable imaging techniques about fusion status are radiographs (conventional plain films, dynamic flexion/extension views), CT, radionuclide bone scans, and MR imaging. Radiography remains the primary modality for routine follow-up, but CT shows hardware position in relation to bone,

Table 3
Main type of spinal instrumentation

Pedicle screws	Used with plates, hooks, or rods Typically used for spinal instability associated with trauma, to promote bony fusion, and for degenerative disease with instability, with or without spondylolisthesis. Optimal screw placement is typically along the medial aspect of the pedicle, without breaching the cortex or entering the neural foramina.
Translaminar or facet screws	Placed in the lamina or the facet joint when posterior elements are intact.
Interbody spacers	These structures are placed in the intervertebral disc space usually after discectomy. Their purpose is to promote fusion maintaining alignment. They may be solid constructions (ramps) or openwork structures filled with bone graft material (cages) and may be used singly or paired (positioned side by side). Good position when the posterior marker, usually radiopaque, is located approximately 2 mm anterior to the posterior edge of the adjacent vertebral body.
Interspinous spacers	Recently introduced, these spacers are inserted between the spinous process through a small incision along the interspinous ligament. They reduce spinal stenosis by restoring height posteriorly, reducing infolding of the ligamentum flavum, and overriding facets.
Harrington rods	The system consists of at least 1 upgoing and 1 downgoing hook, which are usually placed under the respective laminae, and are connected with a rod. Primarily used to correct scoliosis or for trauma.
Cotrel-Dubousset instrumentation	More flexible than the Harrington rod. Indications are primarily correction of scoliosis and kyphosis. Also may be used in selected cases of trauma and for reconstructive procedures in patients with neoplastic invasion of the vertebra.
Hartshill rectangles	Fixation device. Rectangles held in place posteriorly by sublaminar wires that contribute to the structural integrity of the device. Wire fracture is considered a significant finding.

nerves, spinal canal, and vessels, and demonstrates cortical and trabecular bone continuity at fusion sites. The role of MR imaging following fusion is marginal because of absence of signal from bone and image distortion from devices; however, its direct multiplanar imaging ability is useful to define the exact position of the bone graft or cage, as well as to demonstrate bony consolidation in the further course and to show associated pathology in the central spinal canal (**Figs. 8–10**).

In interbody fusion, interbody spacer lucent markers indicate good position of the device if located 2 mm anterior to the posterior edge of the adjacent vertebral body.

When evaluating posterior spinal hardware, pedicle screws deserve attention because of their frequent use and proximity to neural and vascular structures. Optimal screw placement is typically along the medial aspect of the pedicle, when the screw traverses the central portion of the pedicle

and is parallel to the vertebral endplate. The tip of the pedicle screw should approach but not breach the anterior cortex of the vertebral body.[5,6,13,37]

Most common complications in pedicle screws malposition include the following:

- Medial angulation, which may lead to nerve root irritation (more frequent).
- Lateral angulation, which in the cervical spine may involve the foramen transversarium and the vertebral artery.
- Anterior displacement with penetration of the anterior cortex of the vertebral body, butting the aorta.
- Dural, spinal cord, or nerve root injury.
- Implant loosening, often due to osseous resorption around the screw. Loosening of pedicle screws often may be seen on CT as a rim of lucency around the screw threads.[38]
- Hardware fracture or dislodgment with spinal instability and eventually pseudoarthrosis.

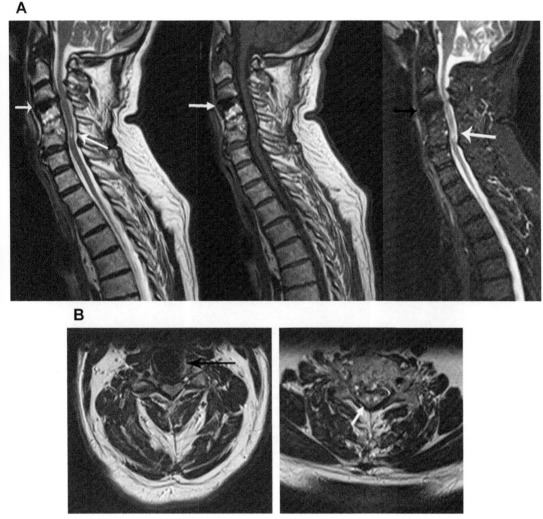

Fig. 8. A 76-year-old patient following cervical C5–C6 discectomy and C3–C4 positioning of interbody cage (*black arrow*). Sagittal T2-weighted, T1-weighted, and STIR (*A*) images, and axial T2-weighted (*B*) images. Note the spinal cord compressive injury at the level C5–C6 (*white arrow*).

The radiologist should also systematically assess the integrity of neural and vascular structures throughout the spine, including the neural foramina, thecal sac, central cord and cauda equina, and foramen transversarium, as well as adjacent structures, such as the major abdominal vessels, psoas musculature, posterior mediastinum, and prevertebral soft tissues.

Teaching points
- In the evaluation of device positioning and integrity, radiography and CT are examinations of choice
- MR imaging is useful especially in patients with neurologic complications and for evaluating spinal cord and paravertebral soft tissue.

POSTOPERATIVE IMAGING AFTER PERCUTANEOUS VERTEBROPLASTY AND BALLOON KYPHOPLASTY

Following percutaneous vertebroplasty and balloon kyphoplasty, imaging comprises the following:

- Baseline imaging at the completion of the procedure;
- Imaging for evaluation of suspected complications due to the procedure;
- Imaging for evaluation of new or recurrent symptoms after initial improvement.

Correct assessment implies awareness of cement changes over time and of the reaction of

A

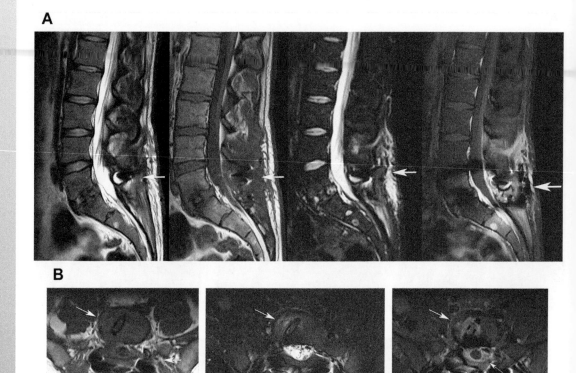

B

Fig. 9. Posterior lumbar interbody fusion in a 27-year-old man treated with pedicular screws at level L5–S1; an interbody cage was also positioned. Sagittal (*A*) and axial (*B*) T2-weighted, T1-weighted, STIR, and contrast-enhanced images show posterior paraspinal fluid collection at the laminectomy site (*white arrows* in *A*) with right neural foramen involvement. Note also the disc changes along the interbody spacer insertion (*white arrows* in *B*). These findings were reported as reactive postoperative changes rather than septic spondylodiscitis. The patient had an improvement of his symptoms and fluid analysis was negative for infection.

the surrounding bone. The first control is made by fluoroscopic evaluation during the procedures, and radiography at its end. Small cement leaks following procedures are inconsequential, but large leaks may cause local or radicular pain, neurologic complications, and pulmonary emboli-zation.[39] Although CT is used to detect main complications, MR imaging shows vertebral and bone marrow changes after vertebroplasty.

MR imaging patterns are mainly characterized by the signal produced by the areas surrounding the cement and by the cement itself. PMMA appears as an oval or rounded intraspongy focal area that is T1 and T2 hypointense with irregular margin (**Fig. 11**); this appearance becomes stable 6 months after treatment. It is surrounded by a T1 hypointense and T2 hyperintense area caused by bone marrow edema; this alteration tends to disappear gradually.

After augmentation, immediate restoration of height and improvement of the wedge angle in

the compressed vertebrae may be seen. In new or persistent back pain after procedures, MR imaging is the first choice to detect new vertebral compression fractures, due to treatment or to the normal evolution of the diseases (osteopenic or metastatic diseases); STIR sequences show intra-spongious edema in adjacent or distant metamer.

PEARLS AND VARIANTS: POSTOPERATIVE IMAGING AFTER PERCUTANEOUS DISC PROCEDURES

Minimally invasive percutaneous techniques for disc herniation, such as chemonucleolysis by plasma light or by radiopaque gelified ethanol (RGE), usually do not require MR imaging follow-up.[40] However, complications, such as intracanal leakage, may occur after RGE injection and must be suspected when a patient presents symptoms suggesting nerve root/spinal cord compression (**Fig. 12**).

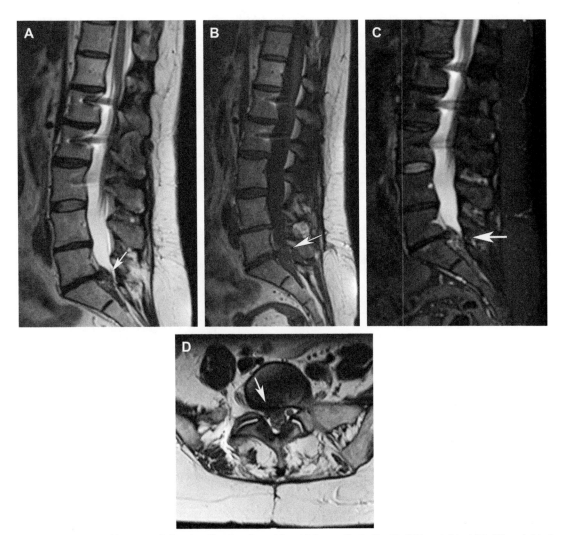

Fig. 10. A 43-year-old woman following fixation from L1 to L5 for scoliosis. Sagittal T1-weighted (*A*), T2-weighted (*B*), and STIR (*C*) images show L5–S1 disc herniation and adjacent intraspinal material, T1-isointense to nucleus pulposus and T2-hypointense, compressing the thecal sac in the laminectomy bed (*arrow*). Axial T2-weighted (*D*) image demonstrates the cauda involvement (*arrow*) and the posterior paraspinal fluid collection. Note the metallic beam-hardening artifacts.

WHAT THE REFERRING PHYSICIAN NEEDS TO KNOW

In the period following an operative treatment of the spine, the referring physician needs to know the following:

- Confirmation of the level(s) treated in comparison with preoperative examinations;
- Interpretation of normal postoperative changes;
- Detection of early/late complications, according to the clinical findings;
- Evaluation of surgical hardware, if present:
  - Interbody implants: 2 mm from posterior margin of the vertebral body;
  - Pedicle screws: centered in the pedicle and aligned with the superior endplate of the vertebral body, with no cortical breach or vascular contact.

SUMMARY

Imaging of postoperative lumbar spine is a common procedure in everyday practice of the radiologist, and a complex task. Knowledge about the clinical presentation of the patients, different types of surgical procedures and instrumentation, normal postoperative changes, and potential complications is essential for proper evaluation.

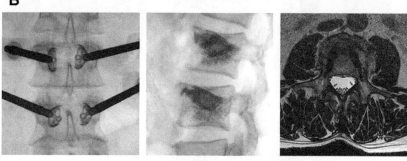

Fig. 11. Preoperative sagittal T2-weighted, T1-weighted, and STIR images (*A*) in a 63-year-old man who presented with L2 and L3 acute vertebral bone fractures and partial collapse of superior endplates with relevant edema of vertebral bodies (*white arrows*) and severe pain under load; patient also had a previous vertebral bone fracture in T12 (*black arrows*). Radiographs (*B*) show percutaneous vertebral augmentation procedure by inserting titanium jack implants into vertebral bodies and injecting mixed biologic and acrylic cement. Posttreatment MR imaging performed after 3 weeks (*C*) showed T1, T2, and STIR-hypointense implants and cement in the vertebral body (*white arrows*), allowing optimal evaluation of hardware positioning. The previous vertebral bone fracture in T12 (*black arrows*) is unchanged. Note that most of the spongious edema in the vertebral body disappeared, and patient's symptoms resolved.

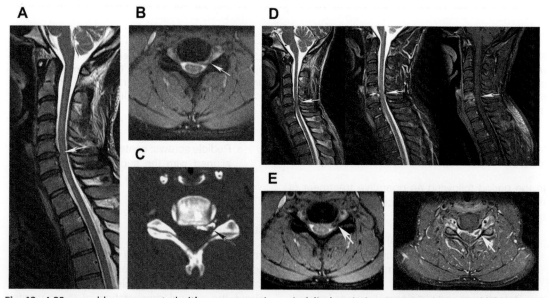

Fig. 12. A 33-year-old man presented with a symptomatic cervical disc herniation. Preoperative sagittal (*A*) and axial (*B*) MR images and CT (*C*) images show the C5–C6 left disc herniation (*arrow*). The patient underwent percutaneous x-ray fluoroscopy-guided injection of RGE. One day after the procedure, the patient presented with new neck pain after an excessive strain. Sagittal T2-weighted, STIR, and contrast-enhanced images (*D*) and axial T2-weighted and fat saturation contrast-enhanced images (*E*) show complete disc material and RGE expulsion, with nerve root and spinal cord compression. Note that there are signs of chemical sterile spondylodiscitis (*arrow*): the nucleus pulposus C5–C6 vertebral bodies appear T2/STIR-hyperintense and show enhancement after contrast injection.

REFERENCES

1. Leone A, Cerase A, Lauro L, et al. Postoperative lumbar spine. Rays 2000;25:125–36.
2. Herrera Herrera I, Moreno de la Presa R, González Gutiérrez R, et al. Evaluation of the postoperative lumbar spine. Radiología 2013;55:12–23.
3. Muto M. Post-operative spine imaging. Abstracts of the 19th Annual Meeting and Exhibition of the International Society for Magnetic Resonance in Medicine, 7-13 May 2011, Montreal, Quebec, Canada. Proc Intl Soc Mag Reson Med 2011;19–23.
4. Jinkins JR. Magnetic resonance imaging of benign nerve root enhancement in the unoperated and postoperative lumbosacral spine. Neuroimaging Clin N Am 1993;3:525–41.
5. Van Goethem JW, Parizel P, Jinkins R. Review article: MRI of the post-operative lumbar spine. Neuroradiology 2002;44:723–39.
6. Rutherford EE, Tarplett LJ, Davies EM, et al. Lumbar spine fusion and stabilization: hardware, techniques and imaging appearances. Radiographics 2007;27:1737–49.
7. Slone RM, MacMillan M, Montgomery WJ, et al. Spinal fixation. Part 2. Fixation techniques and hardware for the thoracic and lumbosacral spine. Radiographics 1993;13:521–43.
8. Vieweg U, Grochulla F, editors. Manual of spine surgery. Heidelberg (Germany): Springer Verlag; 2012.
9. Mathis JM, Barr JD, Belkoff SM, et al. Percutaneous vertebroplasty: a developing standard of care for vertebral compression fractures. AJNR Am J Neuroradiol 2001;22:373–81.
10. Patel VV, Patel A, Harrop JS, et al, editors. Spine surgery basics. Heidelberg (Germany): Springer-Verlag Berlin; 2014.
11. Olsen RV, Munk PL, Lee MJ, et al. Metal artifact reduction sequence: early clinical applications. RadioGraphics 2000;20:699–712.
12. Song KD, Yoon YC, Park J. Reducing metallic artefacts in post-operative spinal imaging: slice encoding for metal artefact correction with dual-source parallel radiofrequency excitation MRI at 3.0 T. Br J Radiol 2013;86:20120524.
13. Willson MC, Ross JS. Postoperative spine complications. Neuroimaging Clin N Am 2014;24:305–26.
14. Suk KS, Lee HM, Moon SH, et al. Recurrent lumbar disc herniation: results of operative management. Spine 2001;26:672–6.
15. McGirt MJ, Eustachio S, Varga P, et al. A prospective color study of close interval computed tomography and magnetic resonance imaging after primary lumbar discectomy: factors associated with recurrent disc herniation and disc height loss. Spine 2009;34:2044–51.
16. Georgy BA, Hesselink JR, Middleton MS. Fat-suppression contrast-enhanced MRI in the failed back surgery syndrome: a prospective study. Neuroradiology 1995;37:51–7.
17. Bundschuh CV, Modic MT, Ross JS, et al. Epidural fibrosis and recurrent disk herniation in the lumbar spine: MR imaging assessment. AJNR 1988;9:169–78.
18. Schinco FP, Ladaga LE, Dillon JD. Distinguishing between scar and recurrent herniated disk in postoperative patients: value of contrast-enhanced CT and MR imaging. AJNR 1990;11:949–58.
19. Groen RJM, Ponssen H. The spontaneous spinal epidural hematoma. A study of the etiology. J Neurol Sci 1990;98:121–38.
20. Gehri R, Zanetti M, Boos N. Subacute subdural haematoma complicating lumbar microdiscectomy. J Bone Joint Surg Br 2000;82:1042–5.
21. Reinsel TE, Goldberg E, Granato DB, et al. Spinal subdural haematoma: a rare cause of recurrent postoperative radiculopathy. J Spinal Disord 1993;6(1):62–7.
22. Barbagallo GMV, Piccini M, Gasbarrini A, et al. Subphrenic hematoma after thoracoscopic discectomy: description of a very rare adverse event and review of the literature on complications. J Neurosurg Spine 2013;19:436–44.
23. Ross JS. Specialty imaging: postoperative spine. 1st edition. Manitoba (Canada): Amirsys; 2012.
24. Richards S. Delayed infections following posterior spinal instrumentation for treatment of idiopathic scoliosis. J Bone Joint Surg Am 1995;77-A:524–9.
25. Diehn FE. Imaging of spine infection. Radiol Clin North Am 2012;50:777–98.
26. Hedge V, Meredith DS, Kepler CK, et al. Management of postoperative spinal infections. World J Orthop 2012;3:182–9.
27. Guyer RD, Collier R, Stith WJ. Discitis after discography. Spine 1988;13:1352–4.
28. Grane P, Josephsson A, Seferlis A, et al. Septic and aseptic post-operative discitis in the lumbar spine –evaluation by MR imaging. Acta Radiol 1998;39:108–15.
29. Van Goethem JW, Van de Kelft E, Biltjes IGGM, et al. MRI after successful lumbar discectomy. Neuroradiology 1996;38:S90–6.
30. Gerometta A, Bittan F, Rodriguez Olaverri JC. Postoperative spondylodiscitis. Int Orthop 2012;36:433–8.
31. Meredith DS, Kepler CK, Huang RC, et al. Postoperative infections of the lumbar spine: presentation and management. Int Orthop 2012;36:439–44.
32. Onik G. Automated percutaneous biopsy in the diagnosis and treatment of infectious discitis. Neurosurg Clin N Am 1996;7:145–50.
33. Nandakumar A, Clark N, Smith F, et al. Two-year results of X-Stop interspinous implant for the treatment

of lumbar stenosis: a prospective study. J Spinal Disord Tech 2012;26:1–7.

34. Szpalski M, Gunzburg R, Mayer M. Spine arthroplasty: a historical review. Eur Spine J 2002;11:S65–01.

35. Khoueir P, Kim KA, Wang MY. Classification of posterior dynamic stabilization devices. Neurosurg Focus 2007;22:E3.

36. Murtagh RD, Quencer RM, Castellvi AE, et al. New techniques in lumbar spinal instrumentation: what the radiologist needs to know. Radiology 2011;260: 317–30.

37. Thakkar RS, Malloy JP 4th, Thakkar SC, et al. Imaging of the postoperative spine. Radiol Clin North Am 2012;50:731–47.

38. Douglas-Akinwande AC, Buckwalter KA, Rydberg J, et al. Multichannel CT: evaluating the spine in postoperative patients with orthopedic hardware. RadioGraphics 2006;26;S97–110.

39. Kulkarni AG, Shah SP, Deopujari CE, et al. Epidural and intradural cement leakage following percutaneous vertebroplasty: a case report. J Orthop Surg 2013;21:365–8.

40. Bellini M, Romano DG, Leonini S, et al. Percutaneous injection of radiopaque gelified ethanol for the treatment of lumbar and cervical intervertebral disk herniations: experience and clinical outcome in 80 patients. AJNR Am J Neuroradiol 2015;36(3): 600–5.

Diagnostic Approach to Pediatric Spine Disorders

Andrea Rossi, MD*, Carola Martinetti, MD, Giovanni Morana, MD, PhD,
Mariasavina Severino, MD, Domenico Tortora, MD

KEYWORDS

• Spinal cord • Spine • Children • Dysraphisms • Myelitis • Myelopathy

KEY POINTS

• Understanding embryologic steps and developmental features is crucial for a correct analysis of MR images in pediatric patients.
• Technical requirements (ie, choice of study protocols, sequences and so forth), must be tailored to address the clinical problem in the rapidly changing environment of the growing pediatric spine.
• Clinical presentations in children with severe, function-threatening disorders can be subtle and long-standing, leading to delays in the diagnosis.
• A working knowledge of the main indications and limitations for spinal imaging in children, including pitfalls or normal variants, is fundamental.

INTRODUCTION

Imaging of the spine and spinal cord is commonly required in the pediatric age group to address a wide array of medical conditions, sometimes presenting in the emergency room. MR imaging has made the diagnosis of these disorders easier, faster, and more accurate, thereby enhancing the possibility of an early and case-tailored treatment, mainly thanks to its multiplanar imaging and tissue characterization capabilities and lack of radiation exposure. Although the MR imaging picture in patients with spinal disorders may appear complicated and puzzling even to experienced observers, a rational approach focusing on a correlation of clinical, embryologic, and neuroradiological data greatly facilitates the diagnosis in most cases. In this article, the principal indications for spinal MR imaging in the pediatric age group are discussed, along with a description of the embryologic steps that lead to the formation of the spine, the main technical issues pertaining to pediatric spinal MR imaging, and a few pitfalls or variants that may simulate disorder.

EMBRYOLOGY

The development of the spine and spinal cord is a highly coordinated phenomenon that begins very early during gestation. It consists of several consecutive steps, which are briefly described here.

During gastrulation, the bilaminar embryonic disc, formed by epiblast (future ectoderm) and hypoblast (future endoderm) is converted into a trilaminar disc because of formation of an intervening third layer, the mesoderm. This process begins by day 14 or 15 when the primitive streak, a stripe of thickened epiblast composed of totipotential cells, appears along the midline of the inferior portion of the dorsal surface of the embryo. The primitive streak has a knoblike cranial termination called the Hensen node. Epiblastic cells start migrating toward the primitive streak and pass inward at the primitive pit, a central depression of the Hensen node, to ingress the interface between the epiblast and the hypoblast; the first cells to ingress displace the hypoblast and form the endoderm, whereas subsequent waves of epiblastic

Disclosure: The authors have nothing to disclose.
Neuroradiology Unit, Istituto Giannina Gaslini, Via Gerolamo Gaslini, 5, Genova 16147, Italy
* Corresponding author.
E-mail address: andrearossi@gaslini.org

Magn Reson Imaging Clin N Am 24 (2016) 621–644
http://dx.doi.org/10.1016/j.mric.2016.04.001
1064-9689/16/$ – see front matter © 2016 Elsevier Inc. All rights reserved.

cells migrate laterally above the endoderm to form the mesoderm. Those cells migrating along the midline of the ectoderm-endoderm interface form the notochord. The notochord is the foundation of the axial skeleton and extends throughout the length of the future vertebral column. From the mesoderm surrounding the neural tube and notochord, the skull, vertebral column, and the membranes of the brain and spinal cord are developed. The notochord is required for the ectoderm to become neural ectoderm and form the neural tube.[1]

Establishment of the neural plate marks the onset of primary neurulation. This process occurs about day 18, when the neural plate starts bending, forming paired neural folds. In the following days, these progressively increase in size and approach each other to eventually fuse in the midline to form the neural tube. According to the traditional zipper model, closure of the neural tube occurs first at the level of the fourth somite (future craniocervical junction) and then proceeds both cephalad and caudad. The cranial extremity of the neural tube (rostral or anterior neuropore) closes at day 30, whereas the caudal extremity (caudal or posterior neuropore) closes at day 31. Closure of the posterior neuropore marks the termination of primary neurulation.[2,3]

The posterior neuropore, that is the caudal extremity of the primary neural tube, corresponds to the 32nd somite (ie, the future third sacral metamere). The segment of the spine and spinal cord caudad to somite 32 is formed by secondary neurulation. This embryologic step begins immediately after completion of primary neurulation and proceeds until approximately gestational day 48. During secondary neurulation, the tail bud, a mass of cells deriving from the caudal portion of the primitive streak, lays down an additional part of the neural tube caudad to the posterior neuropore. This cord segment differs from the one formed by primary neurulation in several ways. Although the primary neural tube results from an upfolding of the lateral borders of the neural plate that join at the midline, the secondary neural tube is formed by an infolding of the neural plate, creating an initially solid medullary cord that subsequently becomes cavitated.[4,5] The fate of the secondary neural tube is to undergo an incompletely understood process of regression, degeneration, and further differentiation, called retrogressive differentiation. This process results in the formation of the tip of the conus medullaris, which contains the lower sacral and coccygeal cord metameres, and the filum terminale, a fibro-connectional structure practically devoid of neural elements. The conus medullaris contains a focal

expansion of the ependymal canal called the terminal ventricle, representing the remnant of the lumen of the secondary neural tube.

The development of the vertebral column proceeds simultaneously with that of the neural tube. At first, the paraxial trunk mesoderm is unsegmented. As development proceeds, epithelial spheres, called somites, are formed and undergo maturation in a cephalocaudal gradient. This maturation leads to dissociation of the epithelial somite, forming the dermatome (dorsal), the myotome (intermediate), and the sclerotome (ventral). The dermatome is located underneath the surface ectoderm. It gives rise to dermal cells for the dorsal moiety of the body. The myotome gives rise to all striated muscle fibers of the body. The sclerotome differentiates into cartilaginous cells of the vertebrae, cells of the intervertebral discs and ligaments, and cells of the spinal meninges. Furthermore, the somite gives rise to endothelial cells. The sclerotome is first located ventrally, and then it spreads to enwrap the entire neural tube forming at its dorsal face the so-called dorsal mesoderm, which will insinuate itself between the neural tube and the surface ectoderm after disjunction. On a next step of differentiation, the sclerotomes divide in half horizontally; the bottom half of one fuses with the top half of another to form the vertebrae. Notochordal remnants between the vertebrae become the nucleus pulposus within the intervertebral disc.[6]

IMAGING PROTOCOLS

Imaging of the spine and spinal cord in the pediatric age group is best accomplished with MR imaging in almost all cases,[7] whereas other modalities play a complementary role in selected indications. Sonography can be used as a valid imaging modalities in newborns and small infants[7,8] but is limited by the degree of ossification of the neural arches of the vertebral columns other than by individual operator expertise. Computed tomography (CT) offers a detailed depiction of the structure of bone, but its use must be weighed against radioprotection issues; in principle, CT should be reserved for the elucidation of specific features and should always be tailored to the minimum possible field of view so as to minimize unnecessary radiation exposure.[9]

A significant issue in pediatric MR imaging in general is the capability of small patients to cooperate long and well enough to obtain quality imaging studies. In general, children may be sufficiently cooperative at age 5 years, although specific conditions, such as acute illness or psychomotor delay, may change this. Younger or severely ill children typically require sedation, which is administered differently according to individual center protocols. Imaging during spontaneous sleep with a feed-and-wrap technique is a viable option in the neonatal period; in our experience, unsedated children weighing 5 kg or less can be studied with this technique, with a yield of greater than 80% technical success. Availability of dedicated rooms for the preparation of patients and subsequent awakening greatly improves the chances of success for imaging small infants without sedation.

Recent technical advancements regarding MR imaging equipment have had a great impact on the possibilities of spinal imaging in children as well as in older age groups. The use of multichannel phased-array coils and applications combining multiple images into a single full field of view have greatly improved the visualization of the entire spine in the sagittal plane, making it possible to acquire whole-spine imaging, including the craniocervical junction and sacrococcyx, in a reasonable amount of time. Scanners of 1.5 T remain the most widely available for clinical MR imaging of children. However, 3-T units have been increasingly used in several centers. Advantages of 3-T MR imaging compared with lower-field scanners include better image quality thanks to a higher spatial and contrast resolution, and improved clinical efficiency thanks to a higher temporal resolution. However, the scanners are more expensive, and various artifacts caused by field inhomogeneity, susceptibility, vascular pulsation, and chemical shift are exaggerated. However, technical adjustments may significantly counteract these setbacks.[10]

Spinal MR imaging should include high-resolution sagittal T1-weighted and T2-weighted images covering the whole spine; in case of indications to the study of a specific segment of the spine, it is also useful to include a whole-spine sagittal view to obtain a panoramic appraisal, to rule out coexisting abnormalities and to correctly number the vertebral levels. Short-tau inversion recovery (STIR) is also extremely useful to detect subtle signal intensity abnormalities of the spinal cord as well as of the osteocartilaginous spine; a coronal acquisition offers the advantage of also scrutinizing the paravertebral regions.[11] Axial sequences on either T1-weighted or T2-weighted imaging are used to study specific regions based on the clinical indications or findings on sagittal images; axial T2-weighted images across lesion areas help to determine the cross-sectional extent of the spinal cord involvement, which is an important element in the differential diagnosis. Optimal slice thickness for these sequences should be

3 mm. High-resolution heavily T2 weighted images, obtainable with different technical modalities (eg, constructive interference in the steady state or driven equilibrium [DRIVE]), provide an exquisite depiction of cord/root/cerebrospinal fluid (CSF) interfaces and are particularly useful to look for subtle structural abnormalities, such as those found in the context of spinal dysraphisms. Whenever indicated, postcontrast images should be acquired in the 3 planes of space; fat-suppression techniques are useful in the study of the spinal compartment, especially regarding the characterization of vertebral lesions. Advanced MR imaging modalities, such as diffusion-tensor imaging,[12] are not yet fully incorporated into clinical practice for spinal studies in children because of significant technical issues and challenges, and are not described in this article.

NORMAL FINDINGS AND PITFALLS

Correct interpretation of spinal MR imaging studies in the pediatric age group requires a firm knowledge of several peculiar features related to the normal growth of the pediatric spine, as well as of a few pitfalls that can be mistaken for disorder.

The normal position of the conus medullaris (**Fig. 1**) is a common element of discussion, especially regarding the possibility of a cord tethering abnormality (discussed later). This position is influenced by the phenomenon of relative ascent of the conus medullaris, which is caused by disparity in the growth of the vertebral column relative to the spinal cord such that, as gestation progresses, the conus medullaris occupies a progressively higher position with respect to the vertebral levels. The period of maximum ascent occurs between 9 and 16 weeks' gestation.[13] There have been various studies in the literature assessing the normal position of the conus both in children and adults; among these, Kesler and colleagues[14] showed in a population of children aged 0.4 to 17 years with brain tumors, studied for the exclusion of leptomeningeal spread, that the tip of the conus was on average at the lower third of L1 and the mode of the distribution was at the L1-2 disc space, with no conus ending below the midbody of L2. Using ultrasonography in neonates, Hill and Gibson[13] showed that the mean position of the conus was midway between the L1-2 disc and mid-L2 body, ranging from T12-L1 to L3, with the modal position being L1-2. Thus, it can be supposed with a good degree of certainty that ascent of the cord after birth is minor. The current position of the International Society of Pediatric Neurosurgery regarding this matter is that

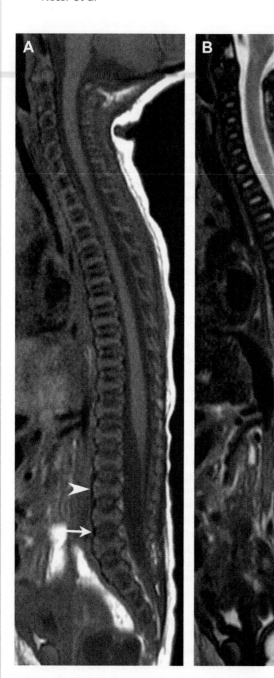

Fig. 1. Normal spine in a newborn. (A) sagittal T1-weighted image; (B) sagittal T2-weighted image. The tip of the conus medullaris lies opposite to the L1-2 disc space. Note, in the T1-weighted image (A), the relative hypointensity of the vertebral centrum (arrow) with respect to the hyperintense intervertebral disc/vertebral endplate complex (arrowhead).

the conus medullaris occupies its adult level, most commonly opposite or cranial to the L1-2 disc space, by birth or at most within 2 months after birth, whereas any conus medullaris lying caudal to the midbody of L2 is to be considered abnormally low and therefore potentially tethered.[15]

Using MR imaging, the assessment of the vertebral level at which any finding occurs (including the position of the conus medullaris) must be done by means of a sagittal sequence that includes the whole spine, from the craniocervical junction to the coccyx. Such images are easily obtainable on state-of-the-art scanners using modern technology, at no significant additional scanning time expense. Some features, especially the presence of transitional vertebrae (more frequently at the lumbosacral junction) or other vertebral deformities (such as unsegmented bars, butterfly vertebra, or hemivertebrae), may impair correct numbering. Inclusion of a coronal scan to count the posterior costal arches may add confidence, although costal malformations may also occur in combination with vertebral anomalies.

In newborns, the normal appearance of the vertebrae and intervertebral discs is markedly different than that of older children and adults[16] (see **Fig. 1**). On T1-weighted images, the central vertebral body has a biconvex shape and appears hypointense because of the prevalent composition in hematopoietic bone marrow; in contrast, the vertebral endplates are still cartilaginous, and appear hyperintense; thus, there is a hyperintense structure, composed of the 2 opposed vertebral endplates and the interposed intervertebral disc, which lies between 2 adjacent vertebral centra. This appearance may be puzzling to unexperienced observers. On T2-weighted images, the disc stands out as markedly hyperintense as opposed to the hypointense appearance of the vertebral body.

The normal sagittal curvature of the spine is also significantly dependent on axial load and, as such, on age (**Fig. 2**). In newborns, the cervical lordosis, thoracic kyphosis, and lumbosacral lordosis are barely visible. The cervical lordotic curve begins to appear as the newborn starts to sustain the head (first 3 months of life); the thoracic kyphosis and lumbar lordosis become progressively more prominent as the child learns to sit, crawl, and eventually stand and walk. In parallel to these events, the thickness of intervertebral discs is uniform in newborns and young children, and the posterior annulus gently and uniformly bulges posteriorly, simulating the appearance of a protrusion. Unlike on sagittal planes, the spine on coronal planes should be straight, and any positioning error should be corrected before scanning proceeds. In the presence of axial load (such as on posteroanterior

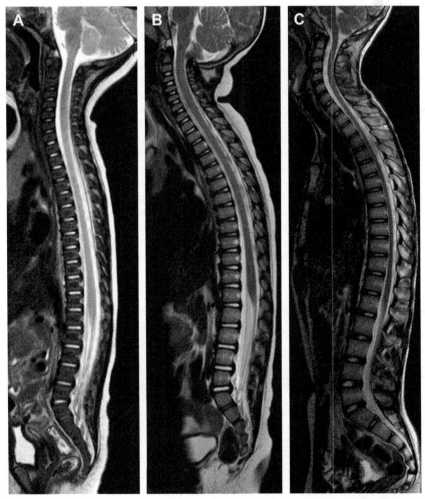

Fig. 2. Normal curvature of the spine. Sagittal T2-weighted images obtained at age 1 (*A*), 6 (*B*), and 18 months (*C*) in normal individuals show progressive appearance of the normal curvatures with advancing age.

radiographs), any deviation greater than 10° in a frontal plane is consistent with a definition of scoliosis, whereas smaller deviations are sometimes termed spinal asymmetries.[17] However, evaluation of the degree of scoliosis is more difficult in the absence of axial load (such as on spinal MR imaging), and caution is advised.

Several other physiologic findings may be prone to misinterpretation. Among common features, injection of perimedullary veins on postcontrast scans can be misinterpreted as a pathologic leptomeningeal enhancement on sagittal scans; recognition of the normal position of the veins on axial planes usually clears the way (**Fig. 3**). Pulsation artifacts generated by CSF in the perimedullary subarachnoid spaces may be prominent, especially in small infants because of their higher cardiac pulsation rate, and may sometimes be mistaken for mass lesions (**Fig. 4**). Normal features may also include visibility of the ependymal canal or terminal ventricle on high-resolution sagittal scans, which should not be mistaken for true hydrosyringomyelia (**Fig. 5**).

MALFORMATIONS

Congenital malformations of the spine and spinal cord (spinal dysraphisms) are usually diagnosed prenatally, at birth, or in early infancy; however, some may be discovered in older children or adults. MR imaging has made the diagnosis of these disorders easier, faster, and more accurate both in the fetal period as well as postnatally, thereby enhancing the possibility of an early and case-tailored treatment, mainly thanks to its multiplanar imaging and tissue characterization capabilities. Classification of spinal dysraphisms requires a balanced correlation of clinical, neuroradiological, and embryologic information. Use of classification schemes may prove helpful in making a diagnosis in everyday clinical practice.[18,19]

Spinal dysraphisms are categorized into open spinal dysraphisms (OSDs) and closed spinal dysraphisms (CSDs).[18,19] The OSDs are characterized by exposure of nervous tissue to the environment through a congenital defect in the child's back; CSDs are covered by skin, although cutaneous birthmarks, such as angiomas, dimples, overgrowing hair, dyschromia, and dystrophy, are often present.[20] Myelomeningocele accounts for most cases of OSD.[18] Clinically, myelomeningoceles are characterized by external exposure and supraelevation of an abnormal, unneurulated segment of the spinal cord (the placode), whereas in the rare myelocele the placode is not extruded (**Fig. 6**). Associated features of OSDs include the Chiari II malformation (in which there is hindbrain herniation through the foramen magnum), hydrocephalus, and complications of myelomeningocele repair.[21–23]

The CSDs are more heterogeneous than OSDs. Some are not clinically evident at birth, and patients are brought to medical attention later in infancy when neurologic complications ensue. Clinical examination is significantly helpful to restrict the differential diagnosis. A critical factor is the presence of a subcutaneous mass on the patient's back. In almost all cases, such mass involves the lumbar or lumbosacral level and is composed of a subcutaneous lipoma. When the lipomatous tissue extends into the spinal canal through a posterior bony spina bifida and attaches to the cord within the spinal canal, a lipomyelocele is diagnosed; conversely, expansion of the subarachnoid spaces with extrusion of the cord-lipoma junction in a posterior meningocele defines a lipomyelomeningocele[18,19] (**Fig. 7**). Other entities presenting with a subcutaneous mass in the

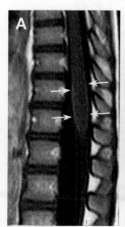 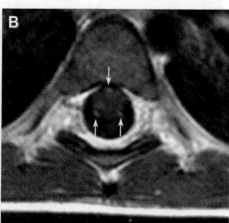

Fig. 3. Vascular injection simulating leptomeningeal enhancement in a 3-year-old boy. (*A*) Gadolinium (Gd)-enhanced sagittal T1-weighted image shows apparent enhancement of the pial surfaces of the conus medullaris (*arrows*), simulating leptomeningitis. (*B*) Gd-enhanced axial T1-weighted image reveals dotlike enhancement corresponding with the anterior and bilateral posterolateral spinal veins (*arrows*).

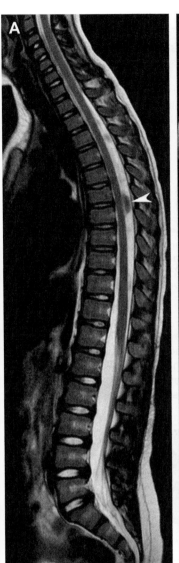
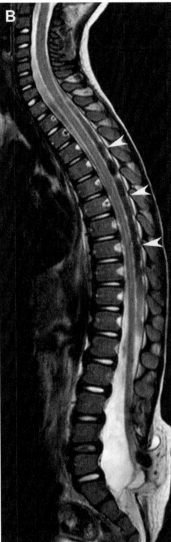

Fig. 4. CSF flow artifacts. (*A*) Sagittal T2-weighted image in a normal 2-year-old boy shows hypointense artifact (*arrowhead*) caused by CSF pulsatile flow in the subarachnoid spaces posterior to the thoracic cord, simulating an intradural mass. (*B*) Sagittal T2-weighted image in an 18-month-old boy with lumbosacral lipomyelomeningocele shows string-of-beads hypointense CSF artifacts (*arrowheads*) posterior to the thoracic cord.

lumbosacral region are meningoceles and terminal myelocystoceles. These entities are extremely rare, especially the latter. While meningoceles are herniations of a CSF-filled meningeal out-pouching, terminal myelocystoceles are characterized by herniation of a hydromyelic cavity that involves the terminal portion of the cord into a meningocele. The CSDs with a tumefaction involving the cervical or thoracic spine are exceedingly rare and are represented by the so-called spectrum of nonterminal myelocystoceles.[24]

Although several birthmarks are associated with various spinal cord malformations, focal hirsutism is significantly associated with diastematomyelia.[18,19] In this entity, there is a variably elongated separation of the spinal cord in two, usually symmetric, halves; these may be contained either within distinct dural tubes separated from one another by a midline osteocartilaginous spur (type I) or within a single dural sac (type II) (**Fig. 8**). Dorsal dimples or ostia can indicate either a dermal sinus or a sacrococcygeal fistula. All fistula openings above the gluteal crease should be presumed to violate the subarachnoid space until proved otherwise.

Patients with caudal agenesis (also known as the caudal regression syndrome) have a heterogeneous constellation of anomalies comprising total or partial agenesis of the caudal portion of the spinal column, anal imperforation, genital anomalies, bilateral renal dysplasia or aplasia, pulmonary hypoplasia, and lower limb abnormalities. An

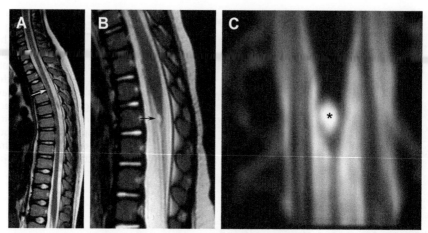

Fig. 5. Incidental spinal cord cavities. (A) In this 10-year-old girl imaged for a suspected lumbar spondylolysis (not shown), sagittal T2-weighted image shows the faintly visible central ependymal canal (*arrows*); this is an incidental finding of no clinical significance. (B, C) In a 2-year-old boy, sagittal T2-weighted image shows small cystic structure at level of the tip of the conus medullaris (*arrow, B*), whereas coronal T2 DRIVE image shows the cyst (*asterisk, C*) in the expected location of the terminal ventricle.

imperforate anus is associated with surgically correctable intradural disorder in at least 10% of patients. The degree of vertebral malformation ranges from isolated agenesis of the coccyx to absence of the sacral, lumbar, and lower thoracic vertebrae; however, most of these anomalies involve partial sacrococcygeal agenesis. The terminus of the spinal cord may be high and abrupt in the most severe cases, whereas it is low and tethered with lesser degrees of vertebral agenesis

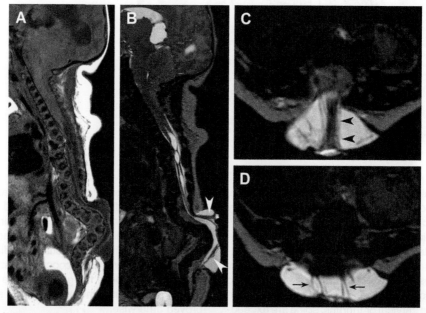

Fig. 6. Myelomeningocele in a 1-day newborn. (A) Sagittal T1-weighted image and (B) sagittal T2 DRIVE sequence show complex malformation consisting of an extruded spinal cord segment within a lumbar meningocele. Note that the T2 DRIVE image, obtained at 0.6-mm slice thickness, is able to provide a better appraisal of the extruded spinal cord (*arrowheads, B*), as well as the thoracic hydrosyringomyelia, with respect to the T1-weighted image, obtained at standard 3-mm thickness. Also note the severe degree of Chiari II and multi-level vertebral abnormalities, with a pronounced focal kyphosis at the level of the dysraphism. (C, D) Axial T2 DRIVE images show extruded spinal cord (*arrowheads, C*) as well as redundant nerve roots coursing within the meningocele (*arrows, D*).

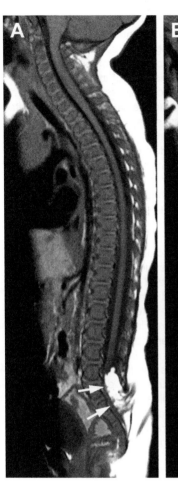 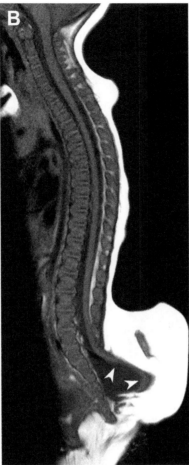

Fig. 7. Differential diagnosis between lipomyelocele and lipomyelomeningocele. (*A*) Sagittal T1-weighted image in a 2-month-old boy with lipomyelocele shows adipose tissue originating from subcutaneous lipoma and extending into the spinal canal (*arrows*) to connect with a low-lying conus medullaris. (*B*) Sagittal T1-weighted image in a 2-month-old with lipomyelomeningocele shows spinal cord protruding out of the spinal canal and into a meningocele (*arrowheads*) where it connects with a huge subcutaneous lipoma.

(**Fig. 9**). Thus, patients with caudal agenesis may be categorized into 2 homogenous groups, characterized not only radiologically but also by different embryology and clinical picture.[25] Patients with segmental spinal dysgenesis, a rare entity embryologically related to caudal agenesis, typically have a protuberance of bony consistence along their back, corresponding with the apex of a kyphotic gibbus at the level of a focal spinal aplasia; they are congenitally paraplegic because their spinal cord is separated into 2 unconnected cranial and caudal portions, with an intervening focal aplastic segment.[26]

The least severe variants of CSD without a subcutaneous mass are represented by tethering abnormalities of the filum terminale, such as the tight filum terminale (a short, hypertrophic filum that produces stretching of the conus medullaris to a low position; ie, below the L2-3 disc space) and filar lipomas (in which fatty transformation of a thickened filum results in a T1 hyperintense stripe on sagittal images). Both these entities may be completely devoid of corresponding birthmarks, and are usually found in patients with sensorimotor dysfunction, muscle atrophy, decreased or hyperactive reflexes, urinary incontinence, spastic gait, or orthopedic deformities that are related to cord tethering.[27]

TRAUMA

The type, severity, and consequences of trauma significantly depend on the peculiar properties of the immature pediatric spine,[28] such as the predominantly cartilaginous composition and the relative mobility and deformability allowed by the laxity of the ligaments. Therefore, vertebral fractures are less frequent than dislocations, ligamentous injuries, epiphyseal detachments, and lesions of the ossification centers. The craniocervical junction is also especially vulnerable in small children because of their comparatively larger heads and weaker neck musculature. Only from about 10 years of age does the more typical adult

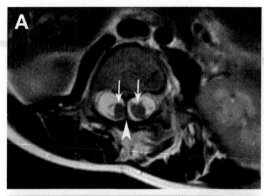

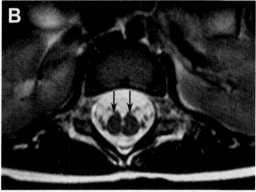

Fig. 8. Diastematomyelia. (A) Axial T2-weighted image in an 8-year-old girl with type I diastematomyelia shows paired hemicords (*arrows*) contained within dual dural sacs, separated by a midline septum (*arrowhead*). (B) Axial T2-weighted image in a 2-year-old girl with type II diastematomyelia shows paired hemicords (*arrows*) contained within a single dural sac, without an intervening septum.

distribution start to prevail, with predominantly cervicothoracic or lumbar injuries. Motor vehicle accidents are the leading cause of spinal trauma in children, followed by sports-related injuries.[29] Patients with craniocervical trauma have a typically acute presentation with neurologic deficit and have a poor prognosis. Intracranial lesions such as hematomas or diffuse axonal injury may coexist and also have a profound impact on the clinical picture and prognosis.

The term SCIWORA is an acronym of spinal cord injury without radiographic abnormality (ie, lacking evidence on either radiograph or CT scan,[30] but evident on MR imaging studies; **Fig. 10**). This form of spinal cord injury is typical of infants and children and is caused by the high mobility and flexibility of the pediatric spine, which allows an intermittent luxation with consequent impact and contusion of the spinal cord. MR imaging usually shows a swollen, T2 hyperintense spinal cord in the affected segment, sometimes with petechial hemorrhages or frank hematomyelia.

Atlanto-occipital and atlantoaxial dislocations are characterized by an anteriorization of the atlas with acute narrowing of the spinal canal, which in turn causes injury to the bulbomedullary junction and spinal cord. This form of injury almost invariably has a severe prognosis, especially when complete ligamentous rupture causes atlanto-occipital dissociation. Less severe forms of progressive atlantoaxial dislocation may occur in patients with inflammatory disorders of the craniocervical junction or with common otolaryngeal conditions, including cervical or tonsillar abscess, pharyngitis, adenotonsillitis, and otitis media, that result in hyperemia and pathologic relaxation of the transverse ligament of the atlantoaxial joint (Grisel syndrome)[31] (**Fig. 11**).

Most vertebral fractures seen in pediatric clinical practice are compression fractures resulting from falls and characterized by wedge-shaped deformity of the involved vertebral body with interruption/fracture of the anterior vertebral margins.[32] More severe fractures include burst fractures, in which both the anterior and posterior contours of the vertebral body are involved, resulting in an intrinsically unstable condition that can further be complicated by intraspinal dislocation of bony fragments with spinal cord damage. Peculiar regional fractures can also be encountered, such as the Jefferson fracture of the atlas and the Anderson and Hangman fractures of the axis. In the lumbar region, the Chance fracture occurs because of flexion-distraction, typically as a result of a seat or lap belt injury, and is intrinsically unstable because it involves all 3 longitudinal vertebral columns. On MR imaging, STIR sequences are especially sensitive to even minimal degrees of bone marrow edema and are helpful to confirm minimal compression fractures, which may sometimes escape detection on conventional radiographs (**Fig. 12**). MR imaging is also mandatory to assess spinal cord damage or intraspinal hematomas in patients with acute neurologic deficit as a result of their trauma.

INFECTIOUS-INFLAMMATORY DISEASES

Acute transverse myelitis (ATM) is a focal inflammatory disorder of the spinal cord characterized by an acute onset of sensorimotor and autonomic dysfunction. Clinical presentation is with pain, paresthesias, leg weakness, and sphincter dysfunction, all of which more or less rapidly progress in the hours to days following the onset. CSF analysis shows pleocytosis or increased immunoglobulin G index. The diagnosis of idiopathic ATM involves exclusion of other causes of acute neurologic involvement, such as

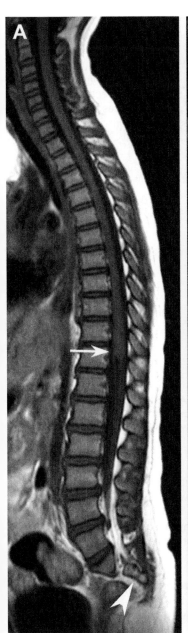
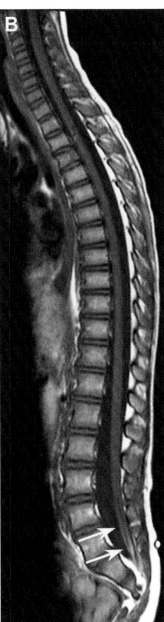

Fig. 9. Caudal regression. (*A*) Sagittal T1-weighted image in an 8-year-old boy with type I caudal regression shows wedge-shaped cord terminus opposite T11 (*arrow*); the last visible vertebra is S1, with an amorphous sacral rudiment below (*arrowhead*). (*B*) Sagittal T1-weighted image in a 2-year-old boy with type II caudal regression shows low-lying conus medullaris, tethered to a short filar lipoma (*arrows*). Note that, counting the vertebrae from C2 downwards, there is complete lumbarization of the first 2 sacral vertebrae (ie, there are 7 lumbar-type vertebrae). Thus, the final visible vertebral rudiment is S4.

extrinsic spinal compression, ischemia, tumor, arteriovenous malformation (AVM), and toxicities.[33] Identified causes of ATM, such as acute disseminated encephalomyelitis (ADEM), multiple sclerosis, and neuromyelitis optica (NMO), must be also be ruled out. MR imaging plays a fundamental role in patients suspected of harboring ATM and should be done emergently, because the presentation of compressive lesions such as extramedullary tumor or hemorrhage can be identical.[34] It is wise to also perform imaging of brain in the same session, in order to promptly identify possible additional lesions (such as those typical of ADEM or multiple sclerosis) while minimizing the need for additional sedation.[34] In idiopathic ATM, MR imaging shows a normal or slightly expanded, T2-hyperintense spinal cord segment involving more than 3 to 4 vertebral levels in length and more than two-thirds of the cross-sectional area. Gadolinium enhancement depends on the degree of inflammation and timing of imaging with respect to clinical onset, and can be absent[29]

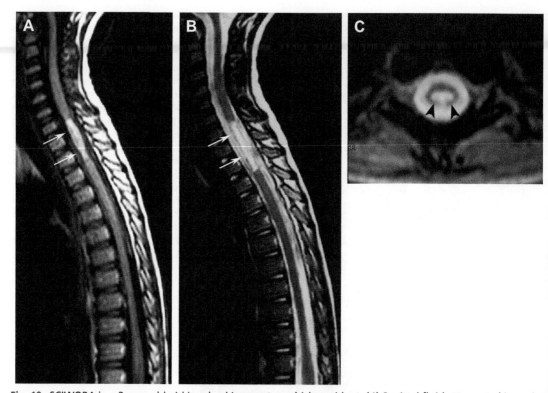

Fig. 10. SCIWORA in a 2-year-old girl involved in a motor vehicle accident. (*A*) Sagittal fluid-attenuated inversion recovery and (*B*), T2-weighted images show intramedullary hyperintense lesion at the C7-T2 level (*arrows*). The osteocartilaginous spine is unremarkable. (*C*) Axial T2-weighted image shows cross-sectional spinal cord involvement (*arrowheads*).

(Fig. 13). Brain imaging is normal in patients with idiopathic ATM. In contrast, in ADEM, MR imaging shows multiple, more or less well-defined or demarcated areas of increased T2 signal intensity both within the cord and in the brain[35]; this is also associated with clinical signs of brain involvement, notably encephalopathy with altered consciousness. Patients with NMO typically have bouts of optic neuritis in conjunction with, or distinct from, their myelopathy attack; they also have typical serologic abnormalities that help in identifying them.[34]

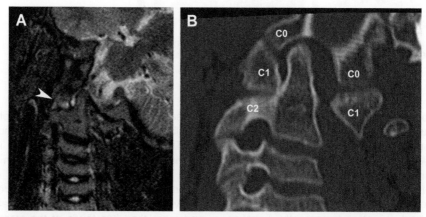

Fig. 11. Grisel syndrome in a 10-year-old girl with prior streptococcal adenotonsillitis and progressive painless torticollis lasting 6 months. (*A*) Coronal STIR image shows severe degree of head tilt; note the hyperintense right lateral mass of C1 consistent with spongious edema (*arrowhead*). (*B*) Coronal reformatted CT scan shows complete loss of coherence between the left lateral masses of C1 and C2, the latter being invisible in this projection.

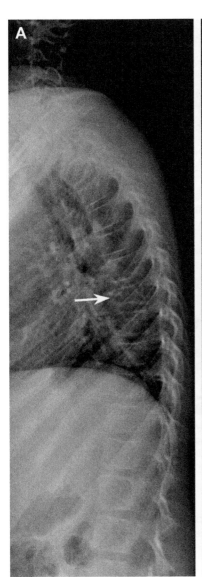 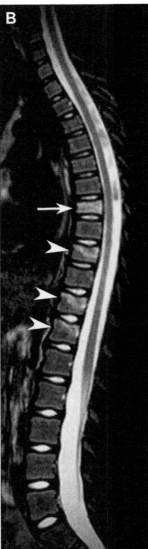

Fig. 12. Compression fractures in a 9-year-old girl who fell while riding a horse. (*A*) Lateral radiographs show compression fracture of T7 (*arrow*). All other vertebral levels appear normal. (*B*) Sagittal STIR image confirm T7 fracture (*arrow*) but also shows subtle signal abnormalities of T9, T11, and T12 (*arrowheads*), consistent with traumatic bone marrow edema.

Spinal cord infection is exceedingly rare in the immunocompetent population; predisposing conditions are usually required for germs to colonize the spinal cord, including congenital heart disease, disorders of the immune system, underlying spinal cord tumors, and especially dermal sinuses,[36] which allow a direct communication between the skin and the CNS. MR imaging shows increased T2 signal intensity and expansion of the cord; more or less well-defined marginal enhancement occurs after gadolinium administration in the case of abscesses. A large part, or even the whole length, of the spinal cord may be involved in the most serious cases (**Fig. 14**).

The Guillain-Barré syndrome (GBS) is an acute inflammatory disorder involving the spinal and peripheral nerves,[37,38] typically presenting after a recent viral disease with lower extremity weakness progressing to flaccid paralysis, often accompanied by sensory disturbances such as pain and paresthesia. CSF analysis shows increased levels of proteins and a lack of inflammatory cells. GBS progresses rapidly, reaching a maximal deficit within 4 weeks of the onset.[38] Unenhanced MR imaging scans are typically unrevealing, because spinal root thickening may be difficult to appraise or even absent. However, gadolinium administration reveals enhancement predominantly of the anterior nerve roots of the cauda

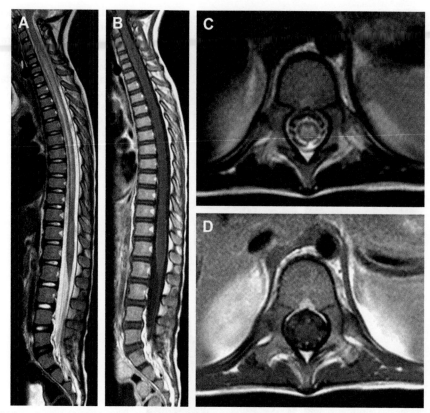

Fig. 13. ATM in a 4-year-old girl. (*A*) Sagittal T2-weighted image shows swollen spinal cord with a hyperintense signal abnormality that extends for much of its length. (*B*) Postcontrast sagittal T1-weighted image shows absent enhancement. (*C*) Axial T2-weighted image shows extensive cross-sectional involvement of the spinal cord, whereas (*D*) postcontrast axial T1-weighted image confirms lack of enhancement.

equina (**Fig. 15**). Involvement of cranial nerves in the same inflammatory process is called Miller Fisher syndrome.[39]

In children, spondylodiscitis can be pyogenic, tubercular (TB), or fungal; infection typically originates in the vertebral body adjacent to the endplate and then spreads to the disc. Patients present with nonspecific findings such as refusal to walk; abdominal pain; fever; and chronic back pain, which is often the predominant complaint. Progression to weakness and paralysis suggests the formation of an epidural abscess with compression of the spinal cord and nerve roots. Abscesses can be particularly large in TB spondylodiscitis, and involve the paravertebral region extensively. On MR imaging, reduction in the height of the intervertebral disc, swelling of the annulus, and T2 hyperintensity of the disc with contrast enhancement are seen in the early stage of the disease. As the disease progresses, loss of integrity of the vertebral endplates is detected (**Fig. 16**). Vertebral collapse can occur, especially in TB cases. Epidural abscesses are frequently

seen, and appear as rim-enhancing lesions in the epidural space.[40]

VASCULAR LESIONS

Spinal cord ischemia is rare in children, and requires a predisposing factor such as cardiovascular surgery, arterial dissection, fibrocartilaginous embolism, or craniocervical instability. Patients experience a strokelike presentation, with signs of acute spinal cord dysfunction that progress to nadir more rapidly than in inflammatory ATM, typically within 4 hours of the onset.[41] The severity of the impairments can vary widely, ranging from paraplegia to minor weakness. On MR imaging, focal or diffuse signal abnormalities are seen (**Fig. 17**); typical anterior spinal artery distributions result in the so-called snake's-eyes appearance on axial T2-weighted images, caused by involvement of the anterior gray horns. Diffusion-weighted imaging (DWI) shows areas of restricted diffusion as in cerebral ischemia; however, implementation of DWI sequences is usually more

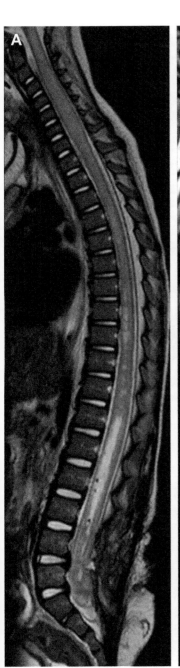
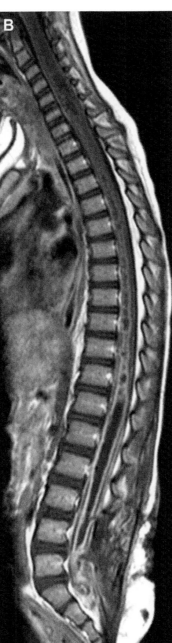

Fig. 14. Diffuse spinal cord abscess in a 2-year-old with prior surgery for lipomyelomeningocele. (*A*) Sagittal T2-weighted image shows diffuse swelling of the whole spinal cord, with signs of cavitation at the lumbar level. The termination of the spinal cord is low because of the pre-existing malformation. (*B*) Postcontrast sagittal T1-weighted image shows diffuse enhancement of the spinal cord, forming a syrinxlike abscess at the T12-L4 level.

cumbersome and less reliable in the spinal compartment than in the brain.[42]

Spinal cord hemorrhage is exceedingly rare in the pediatric age group. Apart from exceptional idiopathic cases, hematomyelia can be caused by bleeding diathesis caused by coagulation imbalance, trauma, or vascular malformations, such as AVMs or cavernomas. AVMs are usually identifiable because of the presence of tangles of dilated vessels forming an intramedullary or pial nidus[43] (**Fig. 18**). Cavernomas are exceptionally found in the spinal compartment; they produce blooming T2* hypointensities because of hemosiderin staining.

TUMORS

Tumors of the spine and spinal cord may present with chronic back pain; however, patients often present in the emergency room despite the

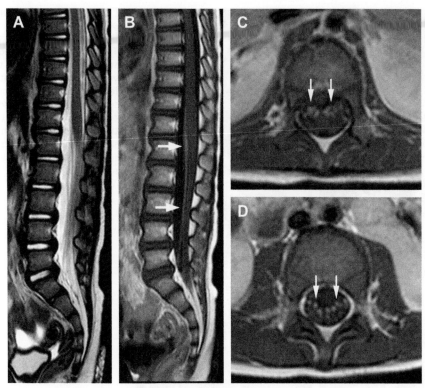

Fig. 15. GBS in a 3-year-old boy. (*A*) Sagittal T2-weighted image is unrevealing. (*B*) Sagittal and (*C, D*) axial post-contrast T1-weighted images show enhancement of anterior nerve roots of the cauda equina (*arrows*).

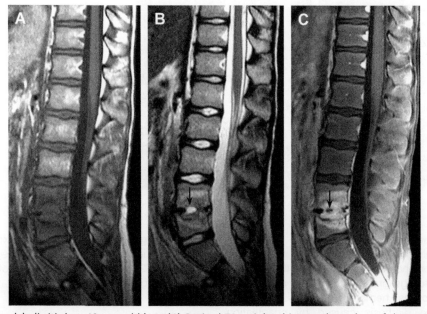

Fig. 16. Spondylodiscitis in a 10-year-old boy. (*A*) Sagittal T1-weighted image shows loss of demarcation of the vertebral endplates at L4-5 and abnormal signal intensity of both vertebrae and intersomatic disc. (*B*) Sagittal T2-weighted image shows that the central disc portion is hyperintense (*arrow*) consistent with necrosis. (*C*) Post-contrast sagittal T1-weighted image shows marked enhancement of the disc, vertebral end plates, and adjacent vertebral bodies. The necrotic disc portion stands out as hypointense (*arrow*).

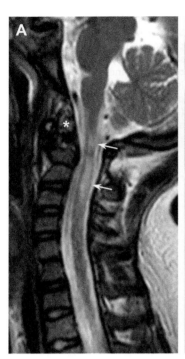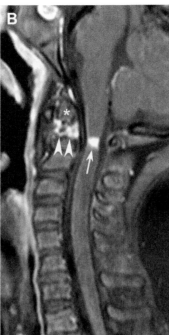

Fig. 17. Spinal cord ischemia in a 7-year-old girl with os odontoideum and cervical instability. (*A*) Sagittal T2-weighted image shows os odontoideum (*asterisk*) and large area of cervical cord edema (*arrows*). (*B*) Postcontrast T1-weighted image shows enhancing soft tissue (*arrowheads*) interposed between os odontoideum (*asterisk*) and dens; there also is focal cord enhancement (*arrow*). Instability with retrograde fibrocartilaginous embolism was presumed to be the cause of spinal cord ischemia. (*Courtesy of* Carlos Ugas, Lima, Peru.)

long-standing duration of their complaints, mainly when additional neurologic deficits related to either compression or infiltration of the spinal cord and nerve roots occur. Spinal tumors are classified according to the involved compartment into intramedullary, intradural-extramedullary, and extradural tumors[44] (**Fig. 19**).

Intramedullary tumors account for 25% of pediatric spinal tumors and prevail in children between 1 and 5 years of age.[44] Astrocytomas (especially pilocytic) are the most common lesion type in children (82% of cases), whereas ependymomas are uncommon outside the setting of neurofibromatosis type 2. The presentation, duration, and course of the disease may be variable. Affected patients may have a prolonged duration of symptoms before a diagnosis is established. Back pain is often the earliest and most persistent complaint; rigidity and contracture of the paravertebral muscles may result from thecal sac enlargement, involvement of adjacent bone, and impairment of CSF dynamics. Progressive scoliosis may cause delays in the diagnosis if underestimated. Head tilt and torticollis, as well as lower cranial nerve palsies with dysphagia, dyspnea, and dysphonia, may represent early signs of cervicomedullary neoplasms because of involvement of the spinal roots of the accessory nerve. Hydrocephalus with increased intracranial pressure rarely represent the clinical presentation of intramedullary tumors because of obstruction of the spinal subarachnoid spaces, CSF seeding, or increased CSF protein content. On MR imaging, intramedullary neoplasms produce enlargement of the spinal cord giving heterogeneous signal intensity on T1-weighted and T2-weighted sequences. They may be solid or associated with cysts, either neoplastic or nonneoplastic, which are better defined after gadolinium administration. They frequently involve a large portion of the cord, spanning multiple vertebral levels in length. Among intramedullary tumors, ependymomas are especially prone to spontaneous hemorrhage, which may cause abrupt clinical presentations.

In the pediatric age group, intradural-extramedullary primitive tumors are the least common variant and are mostly represented by schwannomas and neurofibromas, usually found in patients with neurofibromatosis. A host of other neoplasms, including filar ependymomas, meningiomas, and atypical teratoid rhabdoid tumors, are found occasionally. Clinical features are represented by pain and signs of cord or nerve root compression depending on the location of the mass.[44]

Extradural tumors account for about two-thirds of all spinal tumors in the pediatric age group and may be grouped into bone tumors, tumors of the epidural space, and extraspinal tumors invading the spine. Affected children usually complain with back pain and myeloradiculopathy. Neuroimaging of extradural tumors requires both

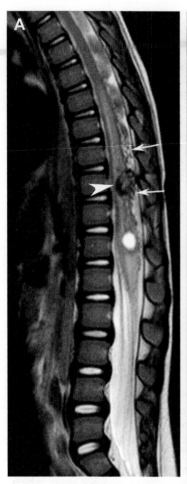
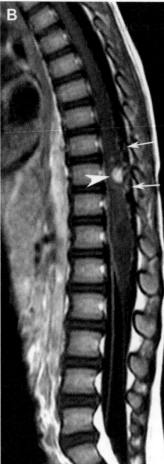

Fig. 18. AVM in a 3-year-old girl. (*A*) Sagittal T2-weighted image and (*B*) postcontrast T1-weighted image show markedly swollen, edematous cord. An aneurysm (*arrowhead*) is noted at T10, associated with diffuse pial venous engorgement (*arrows, A, B*). In addition, there is a focal syrinx at T12.

MR imaging and CT. MR imaging depicts extradural soft tissue components, bone marrow infiltration, and compressive myelopathy compression from the tumor, whereas CT detects the osteolytic or osteosclerotic nature of the lesion and the degree of bone involvement.[44] Among primary bone tumors, osteoid osteomas are often characterized by an acute presentation with nocturnal pain that recedes with nonsteroidal anti-inflammatory medications, and/or with painful scoliosis. Because of the small size of the lesion, accuracy of MR imaging in identification of osteoid osteomas is not high, whereas the typical target appearance is readily shown by CT; however, MR imaging clearly detects the extensive reactive soft tissue masses that are frequently associated with the osteoma.[45] Extrinsic compression of the spinal cord and/or nerve roots is the presenting sign of paravertebral neuroblastoma, the most common non-CNS solid tumor in preschool children. The clinical presentation is variable depending on the location and size of the mass, with neurologic signs appearing with intraspinal extension and thecal sac compression. Neuroblastomas originating from the paravertebral sympathetic chains typically display a dumbbell growth through 1 or more neural foramina, extending a variably sized component into the spinal canal that compresses and displaces the thecal sac and spinal cord. Other extradural tumors causing spinal cord compression include Ewing sarcoma, hematological malignancies, and nerve sheath tumors.[44]

MUSCULOSKELETAL DISORDERS

Many musculoskeletal conditions may present with acute or chronic pain, often resulting in an emergency room presentation.

Arthritis is a heterogeneous group of diseases or conditions that affect the joints, bones, muscles, cartilage, and other connective tissues, hampering or halting physical movement. The most common form in children is juvenile idiopathic arthritis, which, in the spine, most commonly involves the cervical region; symptomatic patients present

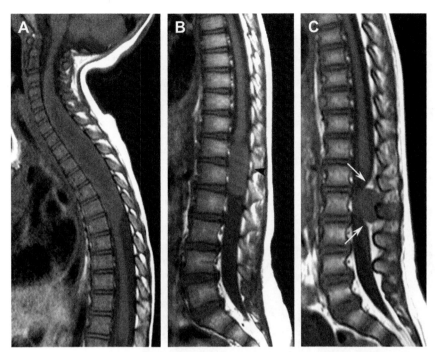

Fig. 19. Spinal tumors: the 3 compartments. (*A*) Sagittal T1-weighted image in a patient with intramedullary astrocytoma shows diffusely swollen cervicothoracic cord. (*B*) Sagittal T1-weighted image in a patient with myxopapillary ependymoma shows intradural-extramedullary mass; note unaffected extradural fat (*arrowhead*). (*C*) sagittal T1-weighted image in a patient with Ewing sarcoma shows extradural soft tissue mass, as indicated by meniscus displacement of the extradural fat (*arrows*).

with pain, stiffness, torticollis, and limited-range head motion. MR imaging reveals synovitis and joint effusion, bone marrow edema, and bone erosions generally involving the C2-3 level. Interruption of the osseous joint surface with signs of inflammation, including hyperintense signal of the interarticular space, synovia, and subjacent bone in STIR images (**Fig. 20**) with corresponding enhancement on postcontrast T1-weighted images is classically found.[46] The dens becomes eroded and may become hypertrophic, causing narrowing of the spinal canal at the craniocervical junction with possible neurologic impairment caused by spinal cord compression.

Disc space calcification (DSC) is a poorly understood, uncommon condition characterized by calcification of the intervertebral disc, usually in the cervical spine. Most patients are boys aged 6 to 10 years who present with local pain or torticollis; intraspinal herniation of a calcified disc fragment may cause acute radiculopathy or sensorimotor signs. DSC is idiopathic, and the course is typically self-limiting so conservative treatment is advocated.[47] MR imaging is especially useful to show associated herniations and the effects on the spinal cord, whereas calcification is less well seen than with CT (**Fig. 21**), which

also reveals irregular endplates with areas of subchondral sclerosis or Schmorl nodes.

Chronic recurrent multifocal osteomyelitis is a sterile skeletal inflammation occurring primarily in childhood and adolescence. The cause is unknown, with autoimmune mechanisms and genetic susceptibility being implicated. The disease has a long, fluctuating course with exacerbations and remissions and presents with pain, rigidity, and malaise. Vertebral involvement is often multifocal, with the thoracic spine being involved most commonly. When present, vertebral collapse may progress to kyphosis and vertebra plana. MR imaging shows osseous edema of the involved vertebrae, well depicted by STIR images, whereas the intervertebral discs are spared. On postcontrast T1-weighted images, enhancement of the involved vertebrae is best appreciated with fat-suppression techniques[48] (**Fig. 22**).

Spondylolysis is a bone defect of the neural arch, usually at the level of the pars interarticularis, caused by repetitive trauma (stress fracture) or dysplasia. Spondylolysis accounts for most cases of low back pain in children older than 7 to 8 years, and is commonly seen in children who practice sports.[49] It is more often bilateral than unilateral and involves L5 in almost all cases. Excessive

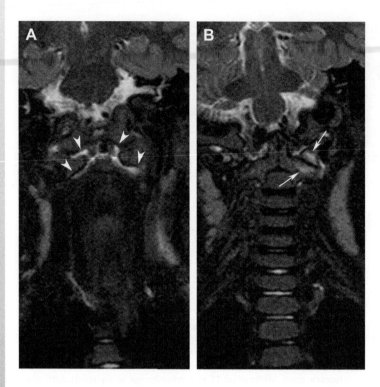

Fig. 20. Juvenile idiopathic arthritis in a 5-year-old girl. (*A, B*) Coronal STIR images show right head tilt as well as redundant fluid collection at C1-2 level bilaterally (*arrowheads, A*); also note subchondral edema at the left C1-2 joint (*arrows, B*).

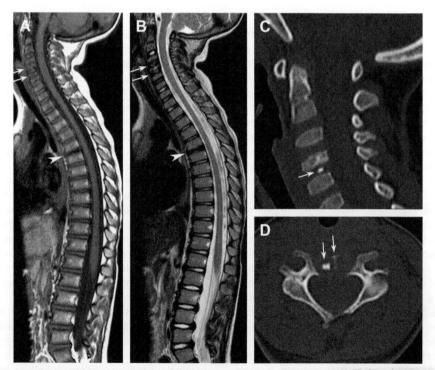

Fig. 21. DSCs in a 3-year-old boy. (*A*) Sagittal T1-weighted image shows ill-defined C3-4 and C4-5 discs (*arrows*) and a hypointense T5-6 disc (*arrowhead*). (*B*) Sagittal T2-weighted image confirms hypointensity of the C3-4 and C4-5 discs (*arrows*), with a hyperintense, collapsed C4 vertebral body; the T5-6 disc is also hypointense (*arrowhead*). (*C, D*) CT scans show DSC at C4-5 (*arrows*); the C4 body is collapsed and irregularly sclerotic.

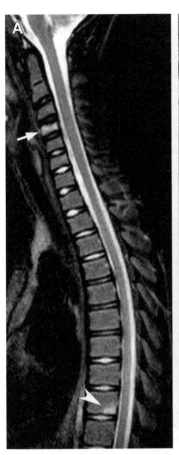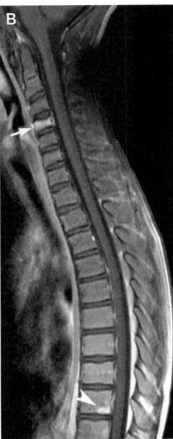

Fig. 22. Chronic recurrent multifocal osteomyelitis in a 12-year-old boy. (A) Sagittal STIR image and (B) postcontrast fat-suppressed sagittal T1-weighted image show collapsed C4 vertebral body, appearing hyperintense (*arrow, A*) and enhancing (*arrow, B*). Note also similar abnormality involving the posteroinferior corner of T9 (*arrowheads*).

motility and instability of the lumbar spine with respect to the sacrum often leads to spondylolisthesis (ie, anterior dislocation) of the involved vertebra. CT shows a thin, irregular interruption of the neural arch at level of the isthmus; sagittal reformats perfectly display the possible associated listhesis. On MR imaging, the defect may not be seen equally well; however, MR imaging is more useful to evaluate associated features, such as osseous edema and redundant masses of inflammatory tissue surrounding the pars defect as well as edema of the spongious bone, that are well seen on STIR images (**Fig. 23**).

Achondroplasia is an autosomal dominant disease with a frequency of 1 in 26,000 live births[50,51] and as many as 80% spontaneous mutations.

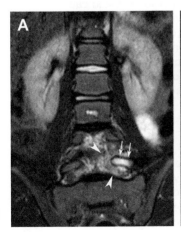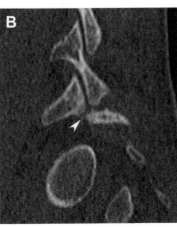

Fig. 23. Isthmic spondylolysis in an 11-year-old girl. (A) Coronal STIR image shows hyperintense left L5 transverse process (*arrows*), consistent with osseous edema; also note soft tissue mass surrounding the involved bone (*arrowheads*). (B) Sagittal reformatted CT image shows pars defect (*arrowhead*).

Clinical manifestations include short-limbed, short-trunked dwarfism with a large head.[52] Newborns with this condition may be hypotonic at birth, possibly as a result of brainstem compression, which may also cause sleep apnea and dysphagia. On imaging, there is a small skull base involving the region of the sphenoid and a small posterior fossa because of underdevelopment of portions of the sphenoid and occipital bones, with a prominent opisthion producing compression of the cervicomedullary structures at the region of the foramen magnum (**Fig. 24**). Spinal canal stenosis is typical and especially involves the cervical and lumbar portions of the canal. The sacrum is horizontalized.

Spondyloepiphyseal dysplasia congenita is an inherited disorder of bone growth caused by mutations in the *COL2A1* gene, resulting in interference with the assembly of type II collagen molecules, which in turn prevents normal development of bone and other connective tissues.[53] In this condition, the vertebrae and epiphyseal centers fail to

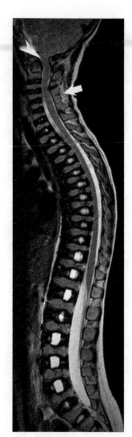

Fig. 25. Spondyloepiphyseal dysplasia in a 2-year-old girl. Sagittal T2-weighted image shows diffuse platyspondyly with significant shortening of the spine. There is stenosis of the foramen magnum (*arrowhead*). Also note fusion of the cervical neural arches (*thick arrow*).

develop, resulting in a short-trunk disproportionate dwarfism with shortened limbs and normal hands and feet; maximum patient height ranges from 0.9 m (3 feet) to slightly more than 1.2 m (4 feet). Kyphoscoliosis and lordosis can become pronounced during childhood, and cause respiratory difficulty; cervical instability may increase the risk of spinal cord damage. On MR imaging, there is diffuse platyspondyly, so the height of the vertebral bodies may approach that of the intervertebral discs (**Fig. 25**). Foramen magnum stenosis with signs of spinal cord damage may complicate the picture.[54]

SUMMARY

MR imaging is the principal imaging modality for studying children with a wide range of spinal and spinal cord disorders, whereas sonography remains a valuable screening tool in children younger than 6 months and CT should mainly be

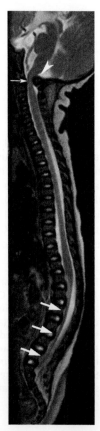

Fig. 24. Achondroplasia in a 4-month-old girl. Sagittal T2-weighted image shows marked prominence of the opisthion (*arrowhead*) with focal cervicomedullary thinning (*thin arrow*). Also note thecal sac narrowing at lumbar level (*arrows*).

used as a second-line confirmatory test for doubtful findings. Knowledge of embryology and developmental anatomy and variations is important for interpreting pathologic images correctly. Technical MR imaging quality must be achieved through correct positioning, use of surface phased-array coils, and use of high-resolution pulse sequences in orthogonal planes. Indications for contrast material administration should be carefully weighed. Cooperation of pediatric patients may not be easily achieved but should be actively pursued in collaboration with the parents or caregivers. Sedation protocols should be available for uncooperative patients.

REFERENCES

1. Corallo D, Trapani V, Bonaldo P. The notochord: structure and functions. Cell Mol Life Sci 2015;72: 2989–3008.
2. Bassuk AG, Kibar Z. Genetic basis of neural tube defects. Semin Pediatr Neurol 2009;16:101–10.
3. De Marco P, Merello E, Cama A, et al. Human neural tube defects: genetic causes and prevention. Biofactors 2011;37:261–8.
4. Catala M. Genetic control of caudal development. Clin Genet 2002;61:89–96.
5. Nievelstein RAJ, Hartwig NG, Vermeji-Keers C, et al. Embryonic development of the mammalian caudal neural tube. Teratology 1993;48:21–31.
6. Scaal M. Early development of the vertebral column. Semin Cell Dev Biol 2015;49:83–91.
7. Sorantin E, Robl T, Lindbichler F, et al. MRI of the neonatal and paediatric spine and spinal canal. Eur J Radiol 2008;68:227–34.
8. Ladino Torres MF, DiPietro MA. Spine ultrasound imaging in the newborn. Semin Ultrasound CT MR 2014;35:652–61.
9. Macias CG, Sahouria JJ. The appropriate use of CT: quality improvement and clinical decision-making in pediatric emergency medicine. Pediatr Radiol 2011; 41(Suppl 2):498–504.
10. Ditchfield M. 3T MRI in paediatrics: challenges and clinical applications. Eur J Radiol 2008;68:309–19.
11. Gupta R, Mittal P, Mittal A, et al. Additional merit of coronal STIR imaging for MR imaging of lumbar spine. J Craniovertebr Junction Spine 2015;6:12–5.
12. Middleton DM, Mohamed FB, Barakat N, et al. An investigation of motion correction algorithms for pediatric spinal cord DTI in healthy subjects and patients with spinal cord injury. Magn Reson Imaging 2014;32:433–9.
13. Hill CA, Gibson PJ. Ultrasound determination of the normal location of the conus medullaris in neonates. AJNR Am J Neuroradiol 1995;16:469–72.
14. Kesler H, Dias MS, Kalapos P. Termination of the normal conus medullaris in children: a whole-spine magnetic resonance imaging study. Neurosurg Focus 2007;23:E7.
15. Ascent of the conus medullaris. In: The ISPN guide to pediatric neurosurgery. Available at: http://ispn.guide/book/ispn-guide-pediatric-neurosurgery. Accessed February 10, 2016.
16. Sze G, Baierl P, Bravo S. Evolution of the infant spinal column: evaluation with MR imaging. Radiology 1991;181:819–27.
17. Van Goethem JW, Van Campenhout A. Scoliosis. In: Van Goethem J, van den Hauwe L, Parizel PM, editors. Spinal imaging. Diagnostic imaging of the spine and spinal cord. Berlin: Springer; 2007. p. 95–108.
18. Tortori-Donati P, Rossi A, Cama A. Spinal dysraphism: a review of neuroradiological features with embryological correlations and proposal for a new classification. Neuroradiology 2000;42:471–91.
19. Rossi A, Biancheri R, Cama A, et al. Imaging in spine and spinal cord malformations. Eur J Radiol 2004;50:177–200.
20. Drolet B. Birthmarks to worry about. Cutaneous markers of dysraphism. Dermatol Clin 1998;16: 447–53.
21. Herman JM, McLone DG, Storrs BB, et al. Analysis of 153 patients with myelomeningocele or spinal lipoma reoperated upon for a tethered cord. Pediatr Neurosurg 1993;19:243–9.
22. McLone DG, Dias MS. Complications of myelomeningocele closure. Pediatr Neurosurg 1991-1992; 17:267–73.
23. Scott RM, Wolpert SM, Bartoshesky LF, et al. Dermoid tumors occurring at the site of previous myelomeningocele repair. J Neurosurg 1986;65: 779–83.
24. Rossi A, Piatelli G, Gandolfo C, et al. Spectrum of nonterminal myelocystoceles. Neurosurgery 2006; 58:509–15.
25. Nievelstein RA, Valk J, Smit LM, et al. MR of the caudal regression syndrome: embryologic implications. AJNR Am J Neuroradiol 1994;15:1021–9.
26. Tortori-Donati P, Fondelli MP, Rossi A, et al. Segmental spinal dysgenesis: neuroradiologic findings with clinical and embryologic correlation. AJNR Am J Neuroradiol 1999;20:445–56.
27. Tortori-Donati P, Cama A, Rosa ML, et al. Occult spinal dysraphism: neuroradiological study. Neuroradiology 1990;31:512–22.
28. Hollingshead MC, Castillo M. Trauma to the spinal column. In: Naidich TP, Castillo M, Cha S, et al, editors. Imaging of the spine. Philadelphia: Saunders/Elsevier; 2011. p. 219–36.
29. Jones TM, Anderson PA, Noonan KJ. Pediatric cervical trauma. J Am Acad Orthop Surg 2011;219:600–11.
30. Pang D, Wilberger JE Jr. Spinal cord injury without radiographic abnormalities in children. J Neurosurg 1982;57:114–29.

31. Bocciolini C, Dall'Olio D, Cunsolo E, et al. Grisel's syndrome: a rare complication following adenoidectomy. Acta Otorhinolaryngol Ital 2005;25:245–9.

32. Huisman TA, Wagner MW, Bosemani T, et al. Pediatric spinal trauma. J Neuroimaging 2015;25:337–53.

33. Scott TF, Frohman EM, De Seze J, et al. Evidence-based guideline: clinical evaluation and treatment of transverse myelitis: report of the Therapeutics and Technology Assessment Subcommittee of the American Academy of Neurology. Neurology 2011; 77:2128–34.

34. Rossi A. Pediatric spinal infection and inflammation. Neuroimaging Clin N Am 2015;25:173–91.

35. Rossi A. Imaging of acute disseminated encephalomyelitis. Neuroimaging Clin N Am 2008;18:149–61.

36. Dev R, Husain M, Gupta A, et al. MR of multiple intraspinal abscesses associated with congenital dermal sinus. AJNR Am J Neuroradiol 1997;18: 742–3.

37. van den Berg B, Walgaard C, Drenthen J, et al. Guillain-Barré syndrome: pathogenesis, diagnosis, treatment and prognosis. Nat Rev Neurol 2014;10: 469–82.

38. Ryan MM. Pediatric Guillain-Barré syndrome. Curr Opin Pediatr 2013;25:689–93.

39. Urushutani M, Ueda F, Kameyama M. Miller Fisher-Guillain-Barré overlap syndrome with enhancing lesions in the spinocerebellar tracts. J Neurol Neurosurg Psychiatry 1995;58:241–3.

40. Sandhu FS, Dillon WP. Spinal epidural abscess: evaluation with contrast-enhanced MR imaging. AJNR Am J Neuroradiol 1991;12:1087–93.

41. Vargas MI, Gariani J, Sztajzel R, et al. Spinal cord ischemia: practical imaging tips, pearls, and pitfalls. AJNR Am J Neuroradiol 2015;36:825–30.

42. Thurnher MM, Bammer R. Diffusion-weighted MR imaging (DWI) in spinal cord ischemia. Neuroradiology 2006;48:795–801.

43. Davagnanam I, Toma AK, Brew S. Spinal arteriovenous shunts in children. Neuroimaging Clin N Am 2013;23:749–56.

44. Rossi A, Gandolfo C, Morana G, et al. Tumors of the spine in children. Neuroimaging Clin N Am 2007;17: 17–35.

45. Woods ER, Martel W, Mandell SH, et al. Reactive soft-tissue mass associated with osteoid osteoma: correlation of MR imaging features with pathologic findings. Radiology 1993;186:221–5.

46. Hospach T, Maier J, Müller-Abt P, et al. Cervical spine involvement in patients with juvenile idiopathic arthritis - MRI follow-up study. Pediatr Rheumatol Online J 2014;12:9.

47. Garg M, Kumar S, Satija B, et al. Pediatric intervertebral disc calcification: a no touch lesion. J Craniovertebr Junction Spine 2012;3:23–5.

48. Falip C, Alison M, Boutry N, et al. Chronic recurrent multifocal osteomyelitis (CRMO): a longitudinal case series review. Pediatr Radiol 2013;43:355–75.

49. Lim MR, Yoon SC, Green DW. Symptomatic spondylolysis: diagnosis and treatment. Curr Opin Pediatr 2004;16:37–46.

50. Rousseau F, Bonaventure J, Legeai-Mallet L, et al. Mutations in the gene encoding fibroblast growth factor receptor-3 in achondroplasia. Nature 1994; 371:252–4.

51. Shiang R, Thompson LM, Zhu YZ, et al. Mutations in the transmembrane domain of FGFR3 cause the most common genetic form of dwarfism, achondroplasia. Cell 1994;78:335–42.

52. Hecht JT, Nelson FW, Butler IJ, et al. Computed tomography of the foramen magnum: achondroplastic values compared to normal standards. Am J Med Genet 1985;20:355–60.

53. Barat-Houari M, Baujat G, Tran Mau Them F, et al. Confirmation of autosomal recessive inheritance of COL2A1 mutations in spondyloepiphyseal dysplasia congenita: lessons for genetic counseling. Am J Med Genet A 2016;170:263–5.

54. Morita M, Miyamoto K, Nishimoto H, et al. Thoracolumbar kyphosing scoliosis associated with spondyloepiphyseal dysplasia congenita: a case report. Spine J 2005;5:217–20.

Index

Note: Page numbers of article titles are in **boldface** type.

Magn Reson Imaging Clin N Am 24 (2016) 645–647
http://dx.doi.org/10.1016/S1064-9689(16)30037-X
1064-9689/16/$ – see front matter

Moving?

Make sure your subscription moves with you!

To notify us of your new address, find your **Clinics Account Number** (located on your mailing label above your name), and contact customer service at:

Email: journalscustomerservice-usa@elsevier.com

800-654-2452 (subscribers in the U.S. & Canada)
314-447-8871 (subscribers outside of the U.S. & Canada)

Fax number: 314-447-8029

Elsevier Health Sciences Division
Subscription Customer Service
3251 Riverport Lane
Maryland Heights, MO 63043

*To ensure uninterrupted delivery of your subscription, please notify us at least 4 weeks in advance of move.

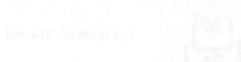

Printed and bound by CPI Group (UK) Ltd, Croydon, CR0 4YY

00/06/2023

01864693-0005